Occupational Therapy

Transition from Classroom to Clinic—Physical Disability Fieldwork Applications

Vicki Smith, OTR/L

Illustrations by David A. Rini, MFA

AOTA The American Occupational Therapy Association, Inc.

Disclaimers

"This publication is designed to provide accurate and authoritative information in regard to the subject matter covered. It is sold or distributed with the understanding that the publisher is not engaged in rendering legal, accounting, or other professional service. If legal advice or other expert assistance is required, the services of a competent professional person should be sought." *From the Declaration of Principles jointly adopted by the American Bar Association and a Committee of Publishers and Associations.*

It is the objective of The American Occupational Therapy Association to be a forum for free expression and interchange of ideas. The opinions and positions expressed by the contributors to this work are their own and not necessarily those of either the editors or The American Occupational Therapy Association.

Anne Rosenstein, AOTA Director of Publications

By Vicki Smith, OTR/L

Edited by Jennifer A. Irey

Designed by Robert Sacheli

Illustrations copyright © David A. Rini, MFA, AMI, Certified Medical Illustrator

Printed in the United States of America.

ISBN 1-56900-003-4

Table of Contents

Dedication i
Preface iii
Special Note to Students v
Editor's Note vii

Chapter 1: Evaluations

Objectives 1
Section 1: Relevance of Medical Chart Information 2
Types of Medical Chart Information 3
- Subjective Information 3
- Objective Information 3
- Assessment Information 4
- Plan Information 4

Medical Chart Review 5
Section 2: Factors That Affect Appropriate Occupational Therapy Evaluation 5
Diagnosis 6
Phase of Recovery 6
Facility Considerations 6
Other Significant Factors 6
Section 3: Alternative Methods of Information Gathering 8
Physician 8
Physical Therapist 9
Speech-Language Pathologist 9
Social Worker 9
Therapeutic Recreation Specialist 9
Registered Dietitian 9
Nurse 9
Case Manager 10

Chapter 2: Treatment Planning

Objectives 11
Section 1: Student Development 12
Stagnation/Unaware Phase 12
Confusion Phase 12
Integration Phase 13
Planning 13

Setting Up Treatment Plans 14
Where is the Patient? 14
What is the Patient's Current Status? 14
What are the Patient's Goals? 14
What Therapeutic Methods are Needed to Reach the Goals? 14
Section 2: Objectives for Effective Goal Writing 15
Verbs 15
Functional Area of Focus 15
Measurable End Point 16
Exploring Communication 17
Patient Reaction to Health Care 18
Communication Parameters 19

Chapter 3: Discharge Process

Objectives 23
Section 1: Health Care Continuum 24
Hospital Services 26
Long-Term Care 26
Rehabilitation Services 26
Outpatient Services 27
Home Health Care 27
Reentry Programs 27
Community Programs 27
Section 2: Home Program Development 28
Chapter Exercises
- Chapter 1 Exercises 31
- Chapter 2 Exercises 83
- Chapter 3 Exercises 121

Exercise Answers
- Chapter 1 Answers 135
- Chapter 2 Answers 173
- Chapter 3 Answers 197

Appendix 1: Abbreviations 207

Appendix 2: Symbols 210

Index 211

Dedication

This book is dedicated to my husband, David A. Smith, and my daughter, Amber Renee Smith. Thank you both for your love and patience.

My sincere thanks to all the students, clinicians, and colleagues who have taught me and inspired the ideas and concepts for this workbook. My special thanks to Vidya B. Kudva, MD, and Sue Hill.

Preface

Students and educators of occupational therapy face many challenges in completing the clinical practicum education requirements for the transition between student and professional. The student can be overwhelmed by the vast amount of information that is introduced during the first few weeks of a clinical practicum and may have difficulty relating classroom skills to actual practice. Fieldwork supervisors often feel that students know very little about the field they have studied for the past 4 years because of the difficulties students have adjusting to actual clinical practice. Therefore, fieldwork educators' goals are to prepare students for the field in order to bridge this gap.

This workbook is designed to aid in the transition from occupational therapy education in the classroom to occupational therapy clinical practice. Its goals are to introduce and reinforce several concepts that are commonly faced in the clinical education process: evaluation, goal writing, interdisciplinary approach treatment planning and delivery, discharge preparation, and situational activity grading. This workbook also introduces the student to the concept of the therapy services continuum available to individuals during the rehabilitation and/or habilitation process.

The introduction of these concepts in the safe environment of the classroom should help decrease student apprehension about the upcoming fieldwork experience. The concepts are also designed to teach students how to develop practical clinical reasoning skills; this should provide fieldwork educators with an education continuum that will prepare students for situations that are similar to those faced in clinical practice.

While the original intent of this workbook was for it to be used solely in the classroom setting, it is evident that many of the exercises and concepts can also be used by fieldwork supervisors to assist students in achieving specific learning objectives. This technique may reduce the anxiety that many students experience during the transition from the classroom to a professional setting.

The workbook has three chapters that are aimed at leading the student through the practical phases of evaluation, treatment, education, and discharge planning. Each chapter begins with objectives that outline the emphasis of the content and concludes with the exercises that are provided at the end of the book. The exercises consist of case descriptions that contain common medical abbreviations, which are itemized and defined in Appendix A. Use of such medical terms allows the student to become familiar with the type of information that he or she will likely encounter in clinical practice. Each case description includes open-ended questions that are designed to lead the student through the clinical reasoning process, and thus relate theory to practice. Throughout the workbook, there are several examples that require ethical considerations, which allow the student to practice forming a professional position that will later prove useful in similar situations.

The student should have his or her exercises evaluated but not graded. Classroom education and fieldwork education have very different student evaluation styles. Grading in the classroom relies on continuous feedback on assignments so that the student can measure his or her progress. Fieldwork education differs in that a patient's recovery provides a measurement of progress. The fieldwork supervisor relies on this standard to evaluate the student.

Therefore, it is suggested that the students not receive a letter grade on the workbook exercises, thus simulating the fieldwork experience. It is recommended that students receive credit for completing tasks, class participation, and discussion. Students who are permitted to evaluate their own work will build self-confidence that will carry over to clinical fieldwork.

Another important feature of this workbook is that it requires students to use resources from their prior class work. This encourages students to integrate the knowledge they have learned in class with research problems that will carry over into actual clinical practice. It should be emphasized that there are no right or wrong answers. The examples and research are designed to help students develop logical clinical reasoning skills and integrate a vast amount of information that will ultimately help patients establish, maintain, or regain their independence.

I hope that this book will provide a framework for educating and preparing the occupational therapy student for fieldwork training. I welcome ideas and comments from colleagues and students; these attributions will help the field of occupational therapy continue to grow and develop with pride.

Special Note to Students

Preparing for clinical affiliation training is a very exciting and anxious time for all students. Classroom studies give students a foundation of information that will assist them with this final education process of becoming a professional. This workbook is designed to give a preview of the types of information and situations encountered within the fieldwork affiliation and in clinical practice. This experience provides a different type of learning than that which is confronted in a classroom setting.

Classroom and fieldwork education are very different. Classroom education is based on continuous feedback provided to the student through grades and evaluations on assignments. In the fieldwork setting, students are given assignments relating to evaluation, treatment, continuing education, theory processing, and practical treatment skills; however, the supervisor does not reinforce these tasks with a grade. The goal of this type of learning is to encourage students to develop self-confidence in their own work and to obtain reinforcement through colleague interaction, patient progress, and self-satisfaction.

Students may need stronger feedback at times to verify that they are meeting the demands of the fieldwork experience. The person to get feedback from is the supervisor. Becoming assertive and asking questions are part of being a professional. Even experienced therapists continue to learn by asking questions of physicians, colleagues, and in some cases, students.

Students often enter their clinical practicum with the impression that they should have learned everything in the classroom setting that will make them effective therapists. Even though the classroom can assist with setting guidelines of theory and practice, no classroom can completely prepare a student to develop patient rapport, engage in treatment processing, interact with colleagues, and cope with other situations that a therapist experiences on a daily basis.

Because human nature and the changing health care system present so many variables to consider in a classroom situation, one of the most challenging and rewarding aspects of being a therapist is learning how to be flexible and creative in dealing with the vagaries of human nature, and medical or facility limitations.

The purpose of the clinical affiliation is to provide students with exposure to these valuable situations but in a setting where guidance is available. The clinical affiliation is a continuation of the education started in the classroom. The student is responsible for the classroom material presented during the occupational therapy education process, and the clinical supervisor is responsible for assisting with the organization of the learned information and the practical aspects of occupational therapy practice.

From the beginning of the occupational therapy education process to professional registration, there are many individuals who play a role in providing the educational requirements needed to become a therapist. Parents, counselors, teachers, school administrators, fieldwork coordinators and supervisors, facility administrators, the American Occupational Therapy Association (AOTA), and the American Occupational Therapy Certification Board (AOTCB), are several examples. Even after a student's formal education is completed, he or she will continue to learn from colleagues, patients, clients, continuing education, students, and practice. This workbook will assist the student in applying the vast amount of information he or she has received over the past few years and making the successful transition from student to clinician.

Editor's Note

Occupational therapists use many terms to describe the individuals who receive therapeutic intervention. *Client* and *resident* are often used to avoid negative stereotypes that may be associated with the term *patient*. However, in an effort to be consistent, this workbook identifies the individuals receiving therapy as *patients* and is not meant to have a negative connotation.

Chapter 1
Evaluations

Objectives

After completing this chapter and the exercises, the student should be able to:

- Identify the types of information found in a medical chart and explore the relevance of the information to an occupational therapy treatment plan.
- Identify four elements that can assist with providing an appropriate occupational therapy evaluation.
- Identify the significance of being aware of medications during an evaluation.
- Identify various methods of gathering evaluation information in order to design an effective treatment plan.
- Begin to use clinical judgment and reasoning skills to evaluate a patient's functional status.
- Identify the meaning of medical abbreviations.

2 Evaluations

Jane is in her second week of clinical affiliation training for occupational therapy. She has been following her supervisor for those 2 weeks. In that time, Jane has been oriented to the department policies and evaluation forms. She has been introduced to occupational therapists, physical therapists, speech therapists, physicians, nurses, the maintenance crew, and other personnel working in the facility. Jane's supervisor has had her observe her patients and a patient evaluation. Her supervisor does everything with such ease and comfort that being a therapist looks very easy. But Jane is worried that she will do something wrong because she cannot remember anything she has read in the past 2 weeks.

At the end of the second week, Jane is assigned a patient. Her supervisor asks her to review the medical chart and determine what information she will need to begin the patient's evaluation. Jane sits down in the busy staff office and is overwhelmed with the request. She goes to the medical chart and starts recording everything she reads.

She sits back and thinks, "There is so much information here. Where do I start? What am I doing here? I don't know enough to do this."

This is a very common situation faced by students in their fieldwork affiliations. The atmosphere of a clinic is very different from a school classroom. The clinic exposes the student to a great deal of distracting information that makes it very difficult to stay organized and retrieve learned facts.

This chapter is designed to alleviate the anxiety of these situations. The exercises for this chapter, which are included at the end of the workbook, provide the student with practical techniques to further develop skills previously learned in retrieving medical chart information, determine appropriate evaluation methods, and learn alternate methods of gathering evaluation information. The exercises are written with common medical abbreviations, which are defined in Appendix A, to familiarize the student with their uses.

Section 1

Relevance of Medical Chart Information

Documentation is a very important part of being an occupational therapist. The therapist is responsible for accurate evaluation, reevaluation, and documentation of a patient. The therapist's notes will be reviewed by other professionals for many reasons. For example, physicians will review the information the therapist provides to assist them with discharge planning. The therapist's notes can also alert the physician to any change in the patient's status and provide documentation that can help support the physician's diagnosis. Together with the other professionals' input and personal medical knowledge, an informed decision can be made about further medical needs and/or placement of the patient.

Other professionals will also benefit from the reports that occupational therapists provide. For example, a dietitian determines if the diet that he or she has prescribed for a patient is adequate. The dietitian may review the therapy reports and determine whether the patient is performing very low- or high-level activities. The diet plan would then be adjusted to accommodate the patient's nutritional needs in relation to the daily activity level.

Insurance companies, quality assurance representatives, utilization review committees, and medicare auditors will also review the therapist's reports to justify the cost of therapy services. A therapist who works well with patients and provides appropriate therapy for their recovery is not effective if reimbursement funds are lost for the health care provider because adequate documentation was not provided, and the charges are sent to the patient because insurance will not cover the cost of services.

It is also critical to remember that the written reports are legal documents. If an unclear statement is made in a report, consider how it would hold up in a court of law. Occupational therapists are legally responsible for what they write and sign.

Types of Medical Chart Information

An occupational therapist should always review a patient's medical information before evaluating the patient. The patient's past medical history should always be included in the initial note format. When a therapist reviews the medical chart, there will be a great deal of information to consider before he or she is able to determine an appropriate evaluation. Every profession and facility has different types of forms for writing evaluations and recommendations. However, there are four types of information that are common to most reports—*subjective*, *objective*, *assessment*, and *plan* (Weed, 1971). Therapists need to understand the differences between these types of information when developing an evaluation and treatment plan for a patient. Therapists are valuable members of any treatment team when they are able to identify and synthesize these types of information.

Subjective Information

The subjective information includes anything the patient states that is pertinent to his or her therapy. It is also anything the patient or patient's family says that cannot be substantiated, verified, or measured. This information is generally written in a narrative form and can include any of the following:

- Patient's complaints of pain or discomfort.
- Prior functioning and living arrangements.
- Statements that may reflect the patient's mental status.
- Patient's statements related to his or her current functioning.
- Statements made by family members that are pertinent to the patient's treatment process.

An example of subjective documentation would be:

> Pt c/o pain in (R) hip. She indicates she lived alone before her fall and took care of herself. Pt states, "It is January 4, 1901," when asked the date. Family members indicate they have been worried lately about her living by herself. Pt indicates she wants to walk.

This information is considered subjective because the patient's and family's perceptions of the reality of what they are reporting may be distorted. Subjective information can be confused because of different types of interpretations.

For example, the above patient's complaints of pain in the right hip may be related to a recent hip surgery , or they may be a result of unfamiliar stretching done during exercises in physical therapy.

The patient indicates she lives alone and takes care of herself. She could mean that she does not have a roommate in the nursing home and can dress, bathe, and take care of her own personal hygiene. However, the staff may be responsible for maintaining her medications and providing meals. In this case, do we really know how she is cognitively functioning?

She states it is 1901. Does this mean she is disoriented? What caused this problem? Has she always been this way? Is her disorientation a result of medications she is taking, or is she neurologically impaired? Perhaps she did not understand the question? Her family has been worried about her lately because she lives alone. Is there a reason to worry, or are they feeling some guilt because they are unable to be with her all the time?

The patient's goal is to walk. Did she walk before, or has this been an unrealistic goal for the past 2 to 3 years? If her current diagnosis is a right lower extremity amputation, is walking a realistic goal? Has she accepted the reality of the amputation? Does she know about, and is she a candidate for, a lower extremity prosthesis?

Objective Information

The objective information includes any of

the formal evaluation or reevaluation testing that has been performed. This also includes information that is received from a reliable source or from accurate testing procedures. Objective information is found throughout the medical chart and is collected in the clinical settings by all of the professionals involved in the individual's care. Objective information can include any of the following:

- General demographics (i.e., age, sex, race, birth date).
- Past medical history. (This information is classified as being received from a reliable source: physicians, social workers, and other professionals.)
- Referring physician and orders from the physician.
- Diagnosis. (This information is based on the physician's objective testing.)
- Standardized tests (i.e., CT scans, x–rays, blood tests, and therapeutic evaluations.)
- Reports on what a patient is physically or mentally doing at the time of an evaluation as reported by a professional staff member. (Example: Able to walk 50 feet with a walker or able to don/doff a shirt with minimal assistance.)

Assessment Information

Assessment information is primarily opinion based on a professional's subjective and objective evaluation results. This information should reflect, summarize, and draw conclusions from the subjective and objective information only. If a conclusion is not supported by the subjective and objective information, it is not a valid assessment.

Assessment information can include any of the following:

- Opinions that are based on the subjective and objective information researched by a professional. If issues are not addressed in the subjective and objective information, they should not appear in the assessment.
- The patient's physical and mental tolerance of treatment.
- A summary of achieved goals or evaluation results. (This includes progress or gains in function the patient has made since the last written report.)
- Potential for continued treatment.
- Recommended areas of focus for treatment.

Plan Information

The treatment plan is the objective intervention that a therapist will be providing and working toward to assist the patient in the recovery process. This plan is based on the information in the assessment portion of the discipline report. The plan information can include:

- Frequency of recommended treatment.
- Long-term goals (LTGs) which are an estimate of where the patient will be functionally at the end of the treatment process and how long it will take to complete the process.
- Short-term goals (STGs), which are specific problem areas that are addressed to form a logical sequence that works toward LTGs.

See Figure 1.1 for a summary of these concepts.

Figure 1.1.
Types of medical chart information.

Subjective:
Information that the patient states that the therapist feels is pertinent to his or her treatment.

Objective:
Information from formal evaluations or reevaluation testing.

Assessment:
Primarily opinion based on professional subjective or objective evaluation results.

Plan:
Objective intervention that a therapist provides and works towards to assist the patient in the recovery process.

Medical Chart Review

It is important for occupational therapists, when reviewing a patient's medical chart prior to treatment, to assimilate all of the information supplied by the various health care disciplines. For example, a physician may establish very different treatment protocols for a diabetic amputee who must have her insulin level checked 4 times per day and who cannot weight bear on her stump for 6 weeks, and an amputee who is placed on a diabetic diet and can weight bear on her stump in 1 week. Or, for example, a social worker may note that a 79-year-old woman, who has a hip fracture, had been living in a nursing home and was totally dependent for her care; the woman's daughter, alternatively, feels that her mother was functioning independently in the nursing home. The therapist must be aware of all of the information in the medical record to be able to assess the reliability of information received from the daughter and to determine how to provide family education appropriately.

■ Practical Application

Do the exercises on pages 31–35. The exercises implement the different aspects of medical charts reviewed in Section 1.

Section 2

Factors That Affect Appropriate Occupational Therapy Evaluation

An occupational therapist is responsible for assessing and evaluating a patient's physical and cognitive functioning to determine an appropriate treatment plan to restore independence. Assessments have several aspects, as illustrated by Opacich (Christiansen and Baum, 1991):

> Assessment is a process by which data are gathered, hypotheses formulated, and decisions made for further action. In occupational therapy, assessment of performance, assets, and deficits guide establishment of therapy goals and interventions. The effectiveness of the selected intervention is determined by subsequent assessment. When incorporated as an integral part of the process, assessment influences clinical reasoning and action. Additionally, assessment may be necessary to substantiate insurance claims, facilitate school placement, determine independent living status, support litigation, document need for a specific program, or establish competence on the job. (p. 356)

The *Uniform Terminology for Reporting Occupational Therapy Services* (Hopkins and Smith, 1983) provides a complete listing of areas a therapist should consider when performing an evaluation. Providing a complete evaluation according to these guidelines can be unrealistic in many cases because of time restraints, lack of the patient's endurance for the testing, or in some cases, insufficient funding to reimburse services. Nevertheless, occupational therapists should provide timely, responsible, and appropriate evaluations that reflect the patient's needs and that do not conflict with external factors that can interfere with patient recovery.

To determine whether an evaluation is appropriate, a therapist needs to consider many factors (see Figure 1.2) including:

- Diagnosis

- Phase of recovery
- Facility that is serving the patient.
- Other significant factors, including discharge plans, funding resources, past diagnoses, and other areas not related to the patient's current diagnosis.

Diagnosis

A patient's diagnosis can be a starting point for determining areas for an appropriate occupational therapy evaluation. The diagnosis indicates areas of disability the therapist should look for.

For example, a diagnosis of a cerebrovascular accident (CVA) indicates that there may be physical, cognitive, and perceptual deficits. Consequently, all these areas should be evaluated when treating a patient with a CVA diagnosis.

A hip fracture diagnosis is basically characterized by physical limitations. The evaluation for a patient with a hip fracture diagnosis should primarily focus on these limitations.

It is important to remember that understanding a patient diagnosis is only a starting point for an effective occupational therapy evaluation. The following factors are of equal importance.

Phase of Recovery

The patient phase of recovery also helps in determine appropriate occupational therapy evaluation areas. A patient in the acute phase of recovery may have limited endurance for activities. Medical precautions or a connection to medical equipment may prevent the patient from participating in a complete evaluation to determine his or her level of independence. A patient in an intensive care unit (ICU) seen 2 days after a CVA may be on a ventilator, intravenous (IV) drips, and an electrocardiogram (ECG) monitor with lines attached to the chest. As a consequence, the patient will not be able to tolerate a complete occupational therapy assessment, and the evaluation must be tailored to fit the needs at the patient's phase of recovery. On the other hand, a patient with a spinal cord injury, who is in a rehabilitation clinic and has been medically stable for 2 weeks, will probably be an appropriate candidate for a complete evaluation, because this type of patient is in a later phase of recovery.

Facility Considerations

The type of facility a patient is in also determines, to some degree, how a therapist should go about an evaluation. Patients in a hospital setting usually have very short lengths of stay and are generally more restricted by their illnesses. A nursing home will also be restricted in the therapy services it can provide because of the limited exposure the therapist has to the patients. Rehabilitation facilities usually have longer lengths of stay for the patients, and the patients are generally medically stable.

For example, if the evaluation and treatment approaches for a head-injured patient in a hospital, nursing home, and rehabilitation clinic are compared, the length of time the patient is seen and the therapy goals will vary. In the hospital, the patient is seen when he or she is medically unstable and only for 1 to 2 weeks. The nursing home may schedule treatment one time per day for 15 to 20 minutes. In the rehabilitation facility, the patient may get as much as 1 1/2 hours of occupational therapy treatment per day for 4 or 5 months.

Given these time restraints, it may be inappropriate to evaluate cooking skills, for instance, during the initial evaluation at a hospital or nursing home. However, a rehabilitation facility would be an appropriate location in which to address cooking activities.

Other Significant Factors

The therapist is responsible for reviewing each patient's previous medical and social history. This information also leads to areas appropriate for evaluation. A patient with a history of confusion and living in a nursing home, and with a current diagnosis of a total hip replacement, will need to be evaluated in different areas than a patient with the same diagnosis who lives alone. Evaluating and teaching lower extremity dressing skills to the confused patient would probably be detrimental to his or her health, because he or she will probably not remember the total hip replacement precautions and may dislocate the hip prosthesis. The patient living independently would be more appropriate for lower extremity dressing evaluation and training, because he or she is alert enough to maintain the precautions, and the training will allow him or her to maintain independence.

Remuneration for services is one of the toughest issues that therapists face when providing recommendations for continued treatment. This issue is a constant source of discomfort for many therapists and other professionals in all types of facilities. Both for profit and nonprofit facilities operate within a financial budget, and there are times when an entire team of professionals can see the potential for recovery in a patient, and yet the funding is not available to continue treatment. There are no words of wisdom that can solve this situation, however, an effective therapist can provide services that may ease the burden of all persons involved. It is important to choose a theoretical basis of treatment that is the most effective for the patient, given funding limitations.

Figure 1.2.
Evaluation factors.

Diagnosis

Phase of recovery

Facility that is serving the patient

Other significant factors
(i.e., discharge plans, funding resources, past diagnoses) and other areas not related to the patient's current diagnosis

Also, it should be noted that the health care system provides many types of access to therapy services. Therapists should explore the discharge recommendation options for continued services. These issues are discussed further in Chapter 3, along with some practical solutions.

■ Practical Application

Do the exercises on pages 37–62. These exercises review the factors that occupational therapists need to consider while evaluating a patient.

Section 3

Alternative Methods of Information Gathering

Medical chart review and determining the logical areas to assess are only part of an effective occupational therapy evaluation. The initial patient interview is also an important aspect. It provides an opportunity to gather information from the patient so that personal needs and desires can be incorporated into a treatment plan. The interview process allows the therapist to establish a clear understanding and purpose of the occupational therapy treatment. It also provides the patient with an opportunity to discuss the situation and to consider ideas for change (Willard & Spackman, 1983). These are essential components of the evaluation and treatment planning process.

Unfortunately, there are times when a verbal interview is not possible. For example, when a therapist is evaluating a patient who is in a coma state, or when the patient has characteristics of dementia or receptive and/or expressive aphasia, this communication technique is not an option. In these situations, nonverbal communication is necessary to develop a therapeutic relationship. Techniques used to establish effective working relationships in these cases are further explained in Chapter 2.

If the patient has impaired communication skills, the therapist will need to use alternative methods to gather information relating to the living situation, personality, interests, and past history. The treatment team and family can be effective sources for this information. Each member of the treatment team gathers specific details that are shared with other team members to formulate an effective treatment plan. The treatment team (see Figure 1.3) generally consists of a physician, physical therapist, occupational therapist, speech pathologist, social worker, recreation therapist, dietitian, nurse, and in some cases, a case manager.

Physician

In many situations, the physician is the team leader. He or she is responsible for evaluating the patient's health and coordinating the rehabilitation process. This process includes a review of the patient's total body system. Orthopedic, neurological, internal, and external functioning of the individual is considered. The physician prescribes and regulates medications and sets precautions and limitations that the patient

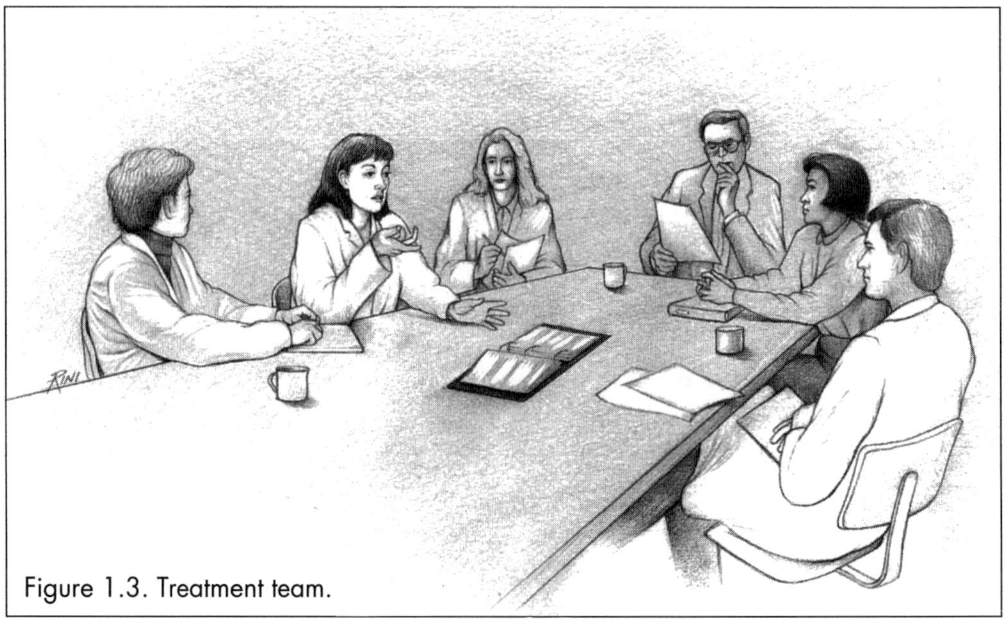

Figure 1.3. Treatment team.

must follow to ensure a safe medical recovery. As a team leader, the physician makes referrals for therapeutic intervention and reviews therapy reports to monitor the patient's physical and cognitive recovery process (DeLisa, Martin, & Currie 1988).

Physical Therapist

The physical therapist provides evaluations for joint range of motion, strength, endurance, and coordination. Assessments also include gross motor skills, sitting balance, standing balance, transfers, and bed mobility. The physical therapist provides training for ambulation, including gait and wheelchair mobility. He or she also uses a variety of modalities, such as superficial and deep heat and cold, hydrotherapy, electrical stimulation, traction, and massage. Many physical therapists provide input for home evaluations and wheelchair equipment recommendations (DeLisa, et al., 1988).

Speech–Language Pathologist

The patient's communication and swallowing abilities are evaluated and treated by a speech–language pathologist. The therapist provides retraining of intraoral deficits that interfere with speech. A management program for the patients with dysphasia is devised. The therapist also provides cognitive reeducation, and evaluation and training for the use of alternative communication devices (DeLisa, et al., 1988).

Social Worker

The primary role of the social worker is to facilitate communication with the patient, family, and rehabilitation team. The social worker's evaluation focuses on the patient's total living situation, including life-style, family, and finances. The goals are to maintain a continuing relationship with the patient and family and to provide assistance throughout the arrangement of an appropriate living situation. The social worker also addresses financial concerns that are related to the impact of the disease or disability on the patient and the entire family (DeLisa, et al.,1988).

Therapeutic RecreationSpecialist

The therapeutic recreation specialist provides treatment intervention that educates patients about leisure activities. He or she provides an assessment that includes the patient's needs, interests, and abilities. This information is incorporated into a program that increases the patient's leisure community access and social skills, and the total spectrum of leisure capacity. The program can include adapted sports, awareness of leisure time and suitable activity choices, education about adaptive equipment that enables the individual to access leisure activities, and assistance for the patient to explore resources for postdischarge activities, such as support groups or community leisure programming (DeLisa, et al., 1988; National Therapeutic Recreation Society, 1992).

Registered Dietitian

The registered dietitian is responsible for managing the patient's nutritional needs. Dietitians assess a patient's nutritional status, develop a care plan that provides the patient with adequate nutritional supplements to facilitate recovery, and monitor the use of all nutritional substances, including intravenous supplements, G-tube feedings, and food substances. The dietitian also provides nutritional counseling and education. As patients' physical activity increases or decreases, their nutritional needs will change. The dietitian monitors these changes and assists with setting restrictions that are medically necessary, such as diabetic diets (Puckett & Miller, 1988).

Nurse

The nurse and the nursing staff are the only members of the team who have the potential to monitor the patients' activity patterns 24 hours a day. As with the other disciplines, the nurse's role varies from facility to facility. The general responsibilities include providing hygiene care, managing medication distribution, watching for medication difficulties, and monitoring environmental factors. These factors include heat, noise, personal property control, sanitation, safety, and infection control. The nurse is responsible for providing interventions that minimize the effects of inactivity, such as repositioning, passive range of motion, and manipulating the environment to avoid sensory deprivation.

The nurse also provides opportunities to integrate various therapy skills into the patient's daily activities. These skills can include use of adaptive equipment for communication, mobility, or self-care. The nurse may also provide opportunities to practice learned skills. The nurse creates an evaluation and treatment plan similar to the other professional disciplines.

Case Manager

Case management is a relatively new discipline that has developed because of the national focus on needing a cost-effective provision of health care services. The National Case Management Task Force Steering Committee (1991) defines case management as "an ongoing process to assure that identified clients of health and human services systems receive appropriate treatment, care, resources, and opportunities to achieve the best and most cost-effective outcome" (*Work summary and survey of case management toward medical case manager certification*, no page number).

There are two types of case managers. One is an internal case manager, who is employed by the facility that is providing services to the patient. The other is an external case manager, who is employed by the payer or funding source for the patient. In some situations, a patient may have both types of case managers.

The role of the case manager is to provide patient advocacy and an objective assessment of an individual's needs and vulnerability by a knowledgeable professional. He or she also provides a goal-oriented plan for the rehabilitation or medical care process and documents the case as it progresses. Case managers maintain communication among the payer, patient, and family regarding any therapeutic recommendations. They coordinate and implement any accepted plan or care to maximize effective use of resources and funds (National Case Management and Task Force Steering Committee, 1991). ▲

■ Practical Applications

Do the exercises on pages 63–82. They emphasize the concepts presented in this section by providing practical situations that students and practitioners experience in the clinical setting.

References

Christiansen, C., & Baum, C. (1991). *Occupational therapy: Overcoming human performance deficits* . Thorofare, NJ: Slack.

DeLisa, J. A., Martin, G. M., & Currie, D. M. (1988). Rehabilitation medicine: Past, present, and future. In J.A. DeLisa (Ed.). *Rehabilitation medicine: Principles and practice* (pp. 7–8). Philadelphia: Lippincott.

Hopkins, H. L., & Smith, H. D. (Eds.). (1983). *Willard & Spackman's occupational therapy* (6th ed.). Philadelphia: Lippincott.

National Case Management Task Force Steering Committee. (1991). *Work summary and survey of case management toward medical case manager certification.* Little Rock, Arkansas: Systematic.

National Therapeutic Recreation Society. (1992). *Therapeutic recreation: A comprehensive approach to a continuum of care.* Alexandria, VA. Author.

Puckett, R. P., & Miller, B. B. (1988). *Food service manual for health care institutions.* Chicago: American Hospital Publishing.

Weed, L. L. (1971). *Medical records, medical education, and patient care* . Cleveland, OH: The Press of Case Western Reserve.

Chapter 2
Treatment Planning

Objectives

After completing this chapter and exercises, the student should be able to:

- Identify guidelines for setting up an occupational therapy treatment plan.
- Initiate the process of writing objective occupational therapy goals and be able to formulate them according to a patient's current status.
- Evaluate and grade activities that reflect treatment goals that progress therapy plans.
- Describe occupational therapy treatment techniques that address a patient's physical and/or cognitive symptoms.
- Relate treatment techniques to occupational therapy theories.
- Identify patient and professional behaviors that interfere with communication.
- Identify effective communication characteristics.

12 Treatment Planning

Larry is in his 5th week of clinical affiliation training at an acute care hospital with a10-bed rehabilitation unit. He has been assigned a couple of patients. He is feeling very good about the evaluations and therapy care he is providing and is beginning to feel like a professional therapist. His supervisor assigned a new patient, George, to his caseload, with instructions to provide a treatment plan outline in a few days. George had a stroke 5 days ago. Larry felt confident in his skills to gather information relating to the evaluation, and he was anxious to provide a thorough treatment plan to his supervisor.

After a couple of days, Larry felt he had enough information to begin the written report and to develop George's treatment plan. As he reviewed the information, he realized that George would need a great deal of skills to become independent in any aspect of self-care.

George's evaluation indicated that he couldn't roll over or sit up. He had problems understanding instructions, his right side was flaccid, and he was severely neglecting the right side of his body. Larry realized that these were the only areas he could address now because George's endurance was still very low. There were a lot of things he didn't know about George's possible deficits. The social worker's report indicated that the family would take him home, and there would be no other discharge considerations. George seemed unprepared for that plan or for any self-care aspects of therapy.

Larry decided to get a candy bar. On the way to the cafeteria, he was thinking about George's situation. "Where do I start? There are so many areas to address in the treatment plan. How do I know if he is going to regain some of his strength, muscle control, or endurance? What are his other deficits that I can't see—like cognitive functioning? How can he possibly go home with his family? Why did my supervisor give me this patient? I am not ready for this, and she should know that. I want to specialize in work hardening; none of this is going to be relevant in that type of clinic."

Section 1

Student Development:

Larry is experiencing a great deal of frustration relating to his position, supervising, and dealing effectively with the new challenges he is facing with George's treatment plan. These are normal reactions that will facilitate the process of becoming a professional.

As with most learning experiences, there is a developmental process for therapeutic competence. The stages of development have been identified as *stagnation* or *being unaware*, *confusion*, and *integration* (Frum & Opacich, 1987). Each stage has specific characteristics that are necessary for a student's development.

Stagnation/Unaware Phase

The phase of development referred to as *stagnation* or *being unaware* generally describes the first few weeks of clinical affiliation. A limited number of skills are displayed by students. These skills tend to be applied uniformly to patients regardless of the diagnosis or the individual patient's situation. This is regarded as an inflexible phase for students because of their limited experience applying theory to the therapeutic process, and interpreting a patient's interactions. During this phase, the student relies heavily on the supervisor for guidance on processes and information.

Two types of student-supervisor relationships can develop. The student may view the supervisor as "knowing all" or having all the right answers. On the other hand, the student may see himself or herself as unable to provide input and fulfill the supervisor's expectations.

Confusion Phase

The *confusion phase* of student development relates to the situation Larry is currently experiencing. It is characterized by feelings of frustration because the student believes he or she possesses limited skills. During this phase of development, students also struggle with appropriate identification of the patient-therapist relationship and being comfortable and versatile with theory approaches. Many students become aware of the need to alter therapy plans to provide effective treatment, but are not able to make these changes effectively.

The student also becomes aware of the tremendous responsibility a therapist possesses when working with a patient. He or she realizes that ethical issues must now be addressed. The student-supervisor relationship also remains a struggle because the student desires independence but still requires guidance from the supervisor.

Integration Phase

The *integration phase* of development is the goal for Larry and his supervisor. This phase is reached when the student has a larger variety of therapy skills and can modify and apply them to different patients and situations. It is also a period when the student is able to understand and deal effectively with personal strengths and weaknesses.

At this point, the student also begins to develop an individual style and technique relating to patient care and professional situations, rather than simply imitating the supervisor. The student is able to establish reasonable and manageable treatment plans and realizes limitations that affect the therapy process, such as facility time constraints and individual patient limitations and values.

Professional judgment begins to develop. This allows the student to handle ethical and legal issues in a variety of situations. The therapeutic relationship conflicts are resolved, which enables effective interaction with a patient regardless of the student's personal feelings. During this phase, the student has a realistic view of the supervisor's strengths and weaknesses. The student may still frequently seek out the supervisor for further in-depth theory and practice knowledge.

These phases of student development are the focus of the clinical affiliation experience. The student is not expected to enter clinical training with all the knowledge needed to provide effective evaluations, treatment, and communication. The fieldwork experience is not a final exam—it is a continuation of training. The most effective way to progress through this process is to communicate with the clinical supervisor.

Planning

Pelland (1987) outlines several aspects important to beginning the therapy planning process, including the need to be aware that a treatment plan continually adjusts during the patient's recovery. The need for adjustments may be related to the individual's recovery pattern or to the alteration of the discharge placement plan.

As indicated in Chapter 1, the anticipated discharge arrangements should help the therapist to identify what skills the individual or family will require. A treatment plan should identify an individual's strengths as well as deficit areas to allow the therapist to provide activities for treatment that use his or her strengths to improve any deficits.

For example, a patient may be very enthusiastic and eager to participate in therapy or may be physically limited but shows good judgment and cognitive functioning. These types of strengths could indicate that the patient is prepared to use an electric wheelchair or other environmental assistance devices.

Finally, a therapist should consider the importance of requesting referrals from other disciplines (Day, 1973; Hemphill, 1982; Hopkins & Tiffany, 1983; Line, 1969; Pedretti, 1985; Trombly, 1989). Today's health care environment requires efficient rehabilitation care. Obtaining information from various disciplines assists in devising a complete therapy plan in an efficient and timely manner. Other disciplines add different perspectives to an individual's physical and mental status that can be an asset to the recovery process and the total treatment plan. This interaction enables the entire team to function together toward mutual goals for the patient's recovery process.

Setting Up Treatment Plans

The process of setting up a treatment plan can be broken down into four sections or questions that identify where the patient is, the patient's current status, the patient's goals, and therapeutic methods to reach those goals. Exploring these areas allows the therapist to combine these facts and formulate a plan that facilitates independence while taking into consideration the facility limitations, the patient's abilities and goals, and the discharge plans.

Where is the Patient?

This question refers to the patient's current situation. Information can include the patient's current diagnosis, past medical history, and age, all of which help determine life-cycle status and current medical precautions. It can also include the patient's previous or current living situation.

The facility situation and prognosis are also valuable considerations when assessing the patient's situation. The combination of this information provides input to past and current physical and cognitive limitations or assets.

What is the Patient's Current Status?

The current status describes the patient's strengths and weaknesses. This information is gathered from the objective testing during an occupational therapy evaluation and from objective reports from other disciplines. Gathering and reviewing objective test information utilizes basic skills that can be enhanced in order to accomplish goals related to the entire treatment plan.

What are the Patient's Goals?

The patient's goals are the major focus of this question. However, other areas also need to be considered. They include family input, discharge placement, and future therapeutic intervention options.

For example, a patient who has suffered a cerebrovascular accident (CVA) and is at an acute care hospital with an average length of stay of 2 weeks, may have a goal of preparing for short-term rehabilitation that has a length of stay from 8 to 12 weeks. Thus, the patient's goal to walk may be unrealistic during the acute hospital stay.

What Therapeutic Methods are Needed to Reach the Goals?

The therapist identifies the major skills that the patient will need to reach the stated goals. These skills become the long-term goals of the treatment plan. The therapist then identifies the specific skills that the patient will need to accomplish long-term goals. These skills become the short-term goals of the treatment plan. The therapist then reexplores the theory options that would fit the situation and outlines therapy activities that address the short-term goals.

■ Practical Application

Complete the exercises on pages 83–94. These exercises are designed to emphasize how a treatment plan varies according to the information that is gathered.

Section 2

Objectives for Effective Goal Writing

The therapy plan outlines the focus areas of treatment and helps the therapist refine the type of theoretical approach used to provide therapy intervention. The therapist does not document the entire therapy plan. The treatment process is tracked through documentation of subjective, objective, assessment, and plan information. This is meant to be a summary or outline of the therapy plan that has been developed. The therapeutic plan consists of long- and short-term goals. These goals should always be reflected in a functional aspect relating to the patient's or family members' abilities.

The purpose of treatment goals is to enhance the understanding of the value of treatment by third party payers, other health care providers, and consumers (Kuntavanish, 1987). *Consumers* refers to the patients and family members who are involved in the occupational therapy process.

A goal should describe the focus of treatment. It should address the functional ability of the patient or family member that the treatment plan is attempting to change, and it should be measurable. A goal can be broken into three components: *verbs*, the *functional area of focus*, and the *measurable end point*.

Verbs

Verbs describe the desired action that the treatment plan is attempting to achieve. They relate to actions performed by the patient or family member, not the therapist. This part of the goal describes the change occupational therapy treatment is expected to produce.

Functional Area of Focus

The *functional area of focus* refers to

Verbs	Functional area of focus	Measurable end point
demonstrate	PROM	Goniometer measurement
strengthen	AROM	Dynamometer
increase	(A)/AROM	Standardized tests
decrease	Hand grip, household mobility	Achieved a functional act: Reach in refrigerator, tolerate w/c positioning
recall achieve perform	UE dressing, LE dressing	Reflects the amount of (A) required to complete tasks: verbal cues, min, mod, max (A)
identify	THR precautions, muscle tone	Muscle testing grading system
list, interpret,recall, apply, use	Any specific muscle or joint, pivot transfers, standing tolerance, sitting balance	Minutes or time number of repetitions
state, classify, construct, describe	W/C mobility, self-feeding, physical endurance, strength	Any method the pt is able to show understanding verbally, in writing, on a computer

Figure 2.1. Functional areas of focus, verbs, and measurable end points.

the skills or activities the treatment plan addresses. These components, which relate to improving function while receiving appropriate therapeutic intervention techniques, can be passive or active.

Measurable End Point

The *measurable end point* indicates the specific desired objective being addressed in the treatment plan. This section can also include the functional aspect of the treatment process.

There are several methods that can be used to document the measurable end point. The chosen method should be as objective as possible and should be used throughout the treatment process.

For example, if the method of measurement for improving upper extremity endurance is the number of exercise repetitions a patient is able to perform during therapy, it should not change to time-related measures. There are examples of verbs, functional areas of focus, and measurable end points listed in Figure 2.1.

The following case study of Bob illustrates the link between the treatment planning process and the development of short- and long-term goals.

Case Study: Bob

Bob has a diagnosis of CVA. His evaluation and tx plan were to be completed within 24 hours. His occupational therapy evaluation results are listed below:

Upper extremity status:
(L) UE ROM and strength are WFL.
(R) UE shows flaccid tone throughout; he has no subluxation, and PROM is WFL; sensation was not tested.

Cognitive status:
Pt able to follow and understand directions. He asks appropriate questions related to recovery. He shows poor ability to sequence skills for dressing.

A	B
LTG: Pt able to perform dressing **STGs:** • Improve UE dressing • Pt demonstrate the ability to cross his legs	**LTG:** Pt demonstrates the ability to dress UEs and LEs c̄ min (A) **STGs:** • Increase UE dressing ability to mod (A) • Improve LE dressing ability to max (A)
LTG: Pt shows improvement c̄ transfers **STG:** • Pt will participate in transfer training	**LTG:** Pt able to perform functional transfers c̄ SBA **STGs:** • Pt will perform tub transfers c̄ tub bench and mod (A) • Pt will demonstrate pivot transfers to even surface c̄ min (A)
LTG: Pt will learn techniques for UE care **STG:** • Pt will do UE self-ROM	**LTG:** Pt will perform UE home program **STG:** • Pt will be able to perform self-ROM c̄ demonstration and handout

Figure 2.2. Bob's case study chart.

Transfer status:
Pt requires mod A x 1 for stand-pivot transfers w/c ↔ mat.

Self-care:
Pt dependent for LE dressing. He requires max A for UE dressing 2° to poor sequencing skills.

Strengths:
- Left side UE and LE are strong and show AROM WFL
- Eager and motivated to work on recovery
- Able to understand and follow directions

Weaknesses:
- Unable to sequence steps for dressing tasks
- Right UE flaccid and PROM WFL no subluxation
- Unable to completely bear weight on (R) LE

Discharge destination:
- Home c̄ wife and 18 y/o daughter
- Wife does not work outside the home.

Major skills needed:
- Transfers—commode, tub and regular chairs
- Dressing skills—UE and LE
- Maintain and/or facilitate (R) UE status

In Figure 2.2, Section A represents examples of poor goal writing. The goals are not consistently stated in terms of the patient performing a functional task. They also do not document a measurable end-point. It would be very difficult to visualize the patient's current abilities or his projected skill development from this treatment plan. However, Section B describes functional projections for the long-term goals and specific task development for each short-term goal. A person reading this treatment plan can clearly see the functional progression to recovery.

Exploring Communication

Sarah is completing her 10th week of clinical affiliation. She has a full caseload and is doing her treatment planning and direct care without much supervision. Sarah is sitting down to complete her weekly notes on the progress and status of each of her patients. As she is organizing her work, she thinks about the different personalities of each of her patients and how they respond to the therapy process.

Debbie is an registered nurse (RN) who suffered a severe stroke. She has difficulty sitting up and eating. Her left side is nonfunctional, and her communication and speech comprehension are poor. But Debbie is the most motivated and energetic patient on Sarah's caseload. She will try anything and she is the type of patient who will always show you something new that she has learned on her own.

Derek is an outpatient who broke his wrist. When the cast was removed, he had limited movement and strength in his nondominant hand and wrist. Each therapy session, Derek emphasizes everything that he cannot do. He has quit work and his wife helps him with dressing and with his hygiene needs. Sarah has made several suggestions to both Derek and his wife that would allow him to return to a more normal daily routine; however, they always convey frustrating descriptions relating to his inability to do anything for himself.

Bob suffered a stroke recently. He had a slight decrease of functional use of his right side. Communication is intact, yet he has a few other minor deficits. Sarah taught Bob to propel his wheelchair the first day of therapy. Bob is extremely grateful. Every chance he gets, he expresses his gratitude for her help and knowledge.

Martha had a hip replacement after falling down a flight of stairs. She had a few other bruises and a couple of cracked ribs. It has been a week, and she is walking around the kitchen, cooking, going on outings with recreational therapy, and is preparing to go home. But she doesn't see any progress with her recovery pattern. Her mood and behavior are the same as the first day Sarah saw her. Regardless of what Sarah says regarding Martha's progress, Martha feels she is not recovering because she is still using a walker.

John was hit by a car and broke his clavicle and left femur. John cannot be classified as motivated or unmotivated—he just does what he is asked to do. He really doesn't offer any of his own opinions to the therapeutic process. John is always making jokes and is often the highlight of the therapy clinic. But yesterday Sarah said her usual "Good morning, John. How are you?" and John burst into tears.

Patient Reaction to Health Care

There are many reasons why patients react differently to the health care process. First of all, the hospital or rehabilitation process has a definite impact on the patient. In addition, the patient's illness causes a great deal of anxiety. The patient may also be concerned about role obligations including family responsibilities, financial issues, and deteriorating of friendships (DiMatteo, 1991).

The patient may experience a loss of control, independence, and privacy. DiMatteo (1991) describes the expected hospital patient role as "cooperative, pleasant, and quiet unless there is an emergency." This expectation has been established by the health care system. Health care professionals generally must have heavy case loads in order to meet cost-effective productivity expectations. They also tend to depersonalize the patients' situations. This is a defense mechanism to protect themselves from the discomfort that may occur from working with patients on a personal level. These factors may lead caregivers to treat all patients the same in a quick and efficient manner, rather than on an individual basis.

For example, suppose that a nurse has 4 patients to work with during her shift. Everyone gets a bed bath between 7:00 a.m and 8:00 a.m. If a patient needs to use the bathroom, and needs assistance, he or she may have to wait for help because the nurse is passing out medications to all her patients. As a result, the patient assigned to this nurse has lost his or her ability to control when to use the bathroom or take a bath. These are not characteristics of poor nursing care; they are characteristics of the health care system.

Different patients react to these situations in different ways. Loss of control can cause anxiety because the patient may develop inadequate expectations, or confusion. Feeling helpless or powerless can also cause anxiety or depression. Some patients react angrily to these situations. Others react with denial, and still others react by developing good patient behavior that can also lead to feeling helpless.

Looking at the research that has explored patients' rationale for accessing health care services can help to explain how and why patients react differently to health care and rehabilitation. The same information can give professional insight into why an individual responds or does not respond to therapeutic treatment.

Some individuals are more likely to notice and attend to a symptom or body disorder than others (Mandler & Kahn, 1960). There are also individuals who will continue with their normal daily routine regardless of any pain or discomfort. In addition, there are individuals who are unable to function with any type of abnormality. A person's self-interpretation of his or her illness can also be related to his or her current situation, stress level, or mood. Any of these factors may indicate to an individual that he or she can attend to the current situation or that other factors in his or her life may appear to be more important.

Patients also interpret symptoms based on several other factors. Prior experience and/or expectations can greatly influence how a person will react to a health problem. A woman, who cared for her mother after a stroke during the last few months of her life, may react differently after she herself suffers a stroke than a woman who has had no contact with a stroke victim.

The interpretation of the seriousness of an illness varies from individual to individual. A young girl with dreams of becoming a model may determine that a facial scar is more important to correct than visual perception and cognitive deficits, all of which have been the result of a car accident.

Finally, what the illness represents to an individual determines how he or she will react. Will the illness label the individual? What are the consequences of the illness? Are there life-style changes or is there a long-term rehabilitation process? What does the individual perceive as the cause of the illness? What is the person's interpretation of the duration and cure for the illness (Lau & Hartman, 1983; Nerenz & Leventhal, 1983)?

An individual's interpretation of the use of the health care system and of rehabilitation can determine behavior traits. In addition, age and gender can cause different reactions to therapy. Men may look at illness and rehabilitation as a weakness. Older adults may be more receptive to illness because it is expected at their stage of life. A person's values, life-style, norms, and cultural interpretations also influence the way he or she will seek and respond to rehabilitation or health care in general (McKinlay, 1972).

Finally, after reviewing complex issues that influence a patient's reaction to the therapy process, therapists should remember that it is possible that the individual may not have any of these reactions. The patient may just be tired, sick, and confused.

The principles and theories of occupational therapy specifically address the losses and frustrations that patients experience during a recovery process. The occupational therapy treatment plan that increases independence at any level can restore an individual's sense of control and self-sufficiency. The therapist should keep these patient reactions to health care in mind when providing treatment. This is essential for maintaining a working relationship with the patient. In a busy clinic or hectic rehabilitation center, a therapist may unknowingly be contributing to the problems that cause a negative patient reaction rather than providing methods to relieve these difficult situations. This reinforces the need to consider the patient's goals for the therapy process. The therapist should also make every effort to help the patient understand the current situation at a level that can be accepted. Patients should be provided with opportunities to make choices whenever possible.

Considering the preceding factors, a therapist can have a difficult time providing the patient with a treatment plan and therapy intervention. Obtaining a patient's complete history can provide some insight into an individual's reaction to his or her current situation. However, it is impossible to learn everything about a person's past experiences, values, and life-style. The primary tool a therapist must rely on for ensuring an effective patient interaction, regardless of these factors, is constant communication.

Communication Parameters

Communication is a very effective medium for assisting a patient through any therapy process. A professional with good communication skills will be able to develop a rapport with most people, regardless of the patients' physical and cognitive deficits. Developing a good rapport helps ensure that the patient will follow the recommendations provided by the professional.

However, there are several factors that interfere with good communication. Poor listening skills are a deterrent. The occupational therapist may be very comfortable planning and providing effective methods of implementing treatment, but he or she may discontinue listening to what is important to the patient.

Part of listening skills is being aware of nonverbal communication that conflicts with the patient's comments. Nonverbal communication includes the patient's eye contact, facial expression, tone of voice, touch, and general body language such as posture and limb movements. These signals may serve as a cue for the therapist to consider more options for gathering information. However, this is difficult to interpret when working with individuals who are physically or cognitively limited.

Listening also includes paying attention to families, friends, and other professionals. For example, suppose a young man is being seen by a therapist. During an initial family education process for his parents and sisters, he asks the therapist to provide information to a male friend. The therapist suggests that the friend attend the family meeting. Very shortly and quietly the patient says, "OK." He breaks eye contact and moves out of the room. Upon further investigation by the therapist, she discovers the patient and friend have a homosexual relationship. The therapist receives a release to be able to provide the friend with information and conducts a separate education session. Effective use of verbal and nonverbal communication allows the patient to trust the therapist.

A major characteristic of effective verbal communication includes being polite. A therapist should introduce himself or herself. If working with a patient with cognitive or memory problems, introductions should take place daily to ensure recognition by the patient. Exchanging pleasant words and making eye contact with the patient are both important. The therapist should be in the patient's visual range (DiMatteo & DiNicola, 1982).

A therapist should also be aware of the use of nonverbal communication gestures. The patient often scrutinizes medical professionals' behavior to discover clues about his or her condition or about what to expect. For example, a patient once confided to her therapist that she was going crazy. The patient said she would hear voices in her room and sometimes people would grab her. The woman said, "I never see them, but I hear them. I can't sleep because I am afraid to close my eyes." The patient suffered from a severe right-sided visual neglect. The therapist discovered the incidents were related to the night nurses who turned the patient in bed and to a technician who came to draw the patient's blood. All of them were unaware of the severity of the patient's visual deficit.

Another major characteristic of effective patient communication is empathy. As previously stated, it is impossible for a therapist to know all the influences and life experiences that affect an individual's behavior during the therapy process. However, an empathetic therapist can help the patient overcome issues related to health care services. Carl Rogers defines empathy as:

> A process that involves being sensitive to another individual's changing feelings and "connecting" emotionally to that other person. Empathy involves a process of "living for a time in the other person's life," entering his or her private perceptual world, and seeing events through his or her eyes. Empathy involves avoiding judgments about what the other is feeling and instead trying to understand fully those feelings from the person's perspective. (DiMatteo, 1991, p. 229)

Empathy takes practice. Being nonjudgmental of another's values is not always easy. But effective use of empathy can enhance the therapeutic process because the patient feels understood and that his or her concerns have been addressed. The patient also feels that he or she has had an active role in the decisions related to the treatment plan. These factors build a positive therapeutic relationship that can ensure successful follow-through with treatment recommendations. ▲

■ Practical Application

Do the exercises on pages 95–120. They are designed to be a continuation of the treatment planning process and to provide an opportunity to practice goal-writing skills. There are also several examples of situations that require communication skills for patients and family members involved with the rehabilitation process. These situations were selected to practice empathy skills when working with patients in realistic situations.

References

Day, D. J. (1973). A systems diagram for teaching treatment planning. *American Journal of Occupational Therapy, 27,* 239–243.

DiMatteo, M. R. (1991). *The psychology of health, illness, and medical care: An individual perspective*. Pacific Grove, CA: Brooks/Cole.

DiMatteo, M. R., & DiNicola, D. D. (1982). *Achieving patient compliance: The psychology of the medical practitioner's role.* New York: Pergamon Press.

Frum, D. C., & Opacich, K. J. (1987). *Supervision: Development of therapeutic competence.* Rockville, MD: American Occupational Therapy Association.

Hammond, D. C., Hepworth, D. H., & Smith, V.G. (1977). *Improving therapeutic communication.* San Francisco: Jossey-Bass.

Hemphill, B. J. (1982). The evaluative process. In B.J. Hemphill (Ed.), *Psychiatric occupational therapy* (pp. 3–12). Thorofare, NJ: Slack.

Hopkins, H. L., & Tiffany, E. G. (1983). Occupational therapy—A problem solving process. In H.L. Hopkins & H.D. Smith (Eds.),*Williard and Spackman's occupational therapy* (6th ed., pp. 89–99). Philadelphia: Lippincott.

Kuntavanish, A. A. (1987). *Occupational therapy documentation.* Rockville, MD: American Occupational Therapy Association.

Lau, R. R., & Hartman, K. A. (1983). Common-sense representations of common illnesses. *Health Psychology, 2,* 167–185.

Line, J. (1969). Case method as a scientific form of clinical thinking. *American Journal of Occupational Therapy, 23,* 308–313.

Mandler, G., & Kahn, M. (1960). Discrimination of changes in heart rate: Two unsuccessful attempts. *Journal of the Experimental Analysis of Behavior, 3,* 21–25.

McKinlay, J. B. (1972). Some approaches and problems in the study of the use of services: An overview. *Journal of Health and Social Behavior, 13,* 115–152.

Nerenz, D. R., & Leventhal, H. (1983). Self-regulation theory in chronic illness. In T.G. Burish & L.A. Bradley (Eds.), *Coping with chronic disease: Research and applications* (pp. 13–38). New York: Academic Press.

Pedretti, L.W. (1985). Treatment planning. In L.W. Pedretti (Ed.), *Occupational therapy* (2nd ed., pp. 22–29). Princeton, NJ: Mosely.

Pelland, M.J. (1987). A conceptual model for the instruction and supervision of treatment planning. *American Journal of Occupation Therapy, 41,* 351–359.

Purtillo, R. (1990). *Health professional and patient interaction.* Philadelphia: Saunders.

Trombly, C.A. (1989). The treatment planning process. In C.A. Trombly (Ed.), *Occupational therapy for physical dysfunction* (2nd ed., p. 3011). Baltimore: Williams & Wilkins.

Chapter 3
Discharge Process

Objectives

After completing this chapter and the exercises, the student should be able to:

- Identify discharge settings and compare the levels of services offered at each.
- Provide continued therapy recommendations according to an individual's discharge placement.
- Identify characteristics of home-program development.

24 Discharge Process

Nancy is an occupational therapy student completing her final affiliation. She has been working with Joe for 3 weeks since he suffered a subdural hematoma. During this time, he was making good progress in regaining his independence.

When Nancy first started seeing Joe, there was no indication of how long he would be hospitalized. Nancy was positive about their working relationship and the treatment plan. During the weekly team meetings organized to review Joe's total treatment plan, the social worker reported that Joe would be discharged home by the end of the month, which was in 2 weeks.

After the meeting, Nancy reviewed Joe's treatment plan with the new discharge information to make adjustments. Nancy's treatment focus had been primarily based on neurodevelopmental theory to facilitate Joe's upper extremity recovery and gross motor skills. Her treatment methods had been effective, but the neurodevelopmental therapy process would not be completed in the remaining 2 weeks to enable Joe to go home safely.

As Nancy continued to review the treatment options that would allow her to meet the time restraints, she began to feel that the discharge plan was unfair to Joe in terms of his rehabilitation process. Every treatment option she examined made her feel like she was putting a bandage on Joe's deficits rather than progressing him to his fullest potential of recovery. Nancy feared that once Joe was discharged from the facility, his rehabilitation would stop and he would lose his current level of functioning.

Therapists are taught to see the potential of individuals during the therapeutic process. Their entire education focuses on the evaluation of a patient's potential for independence at all levels of functioning. Nancy found Joe's potential and had been working with him to help him recover his independence. But there are many external factors that influence the recovery process.

A number of these factors have been reviewed in the first two chapters of this workbook. Because of these factors, a therapist may often feel that a patient is not receiving the full benefit of therapeutic recovery. Many times the therapist may feel that if patients do not receive treatment from the therapist's clinic, they will have no chance of recovery.

Section 1

Health Care Continuum

The entire health care services environment has a great deal of influence on a person's rehabilitation and recovery process. Access to and use of health care services is constantly changing. Today's health care environment is particularly dynamic because of the nationwide focus on reducing cost.

Health care should be viewed as a continuum of services that provides support for individuals recovering from an illness or readapting to community and life roles. The occupational therapy services delivery model designed by Baum (Christiansen & Baum, 1991) provides a description of the levels of occupational therapy services that are commonly provided by today's health care system. Figure 3.1 expands on the average service definitions for occupational therapy service. Understanding the basic services that are provided, funding and regulation issues, and the average length of rehabilitation services in health care programs can help the therapist be part of the health care continuum and provide effective discharge recommendations for patients.

As illustrated in Figure 3.1, an individual generally enters the health care system through the hospital or other medical service. The patient can then continue on to a rehabilitation facility, or long-term care, or return home with supportive therapy.

Patients who return home can receive services through outpatient therapy, home health, reentry, or community programs. Patients who return home also often receive an informal

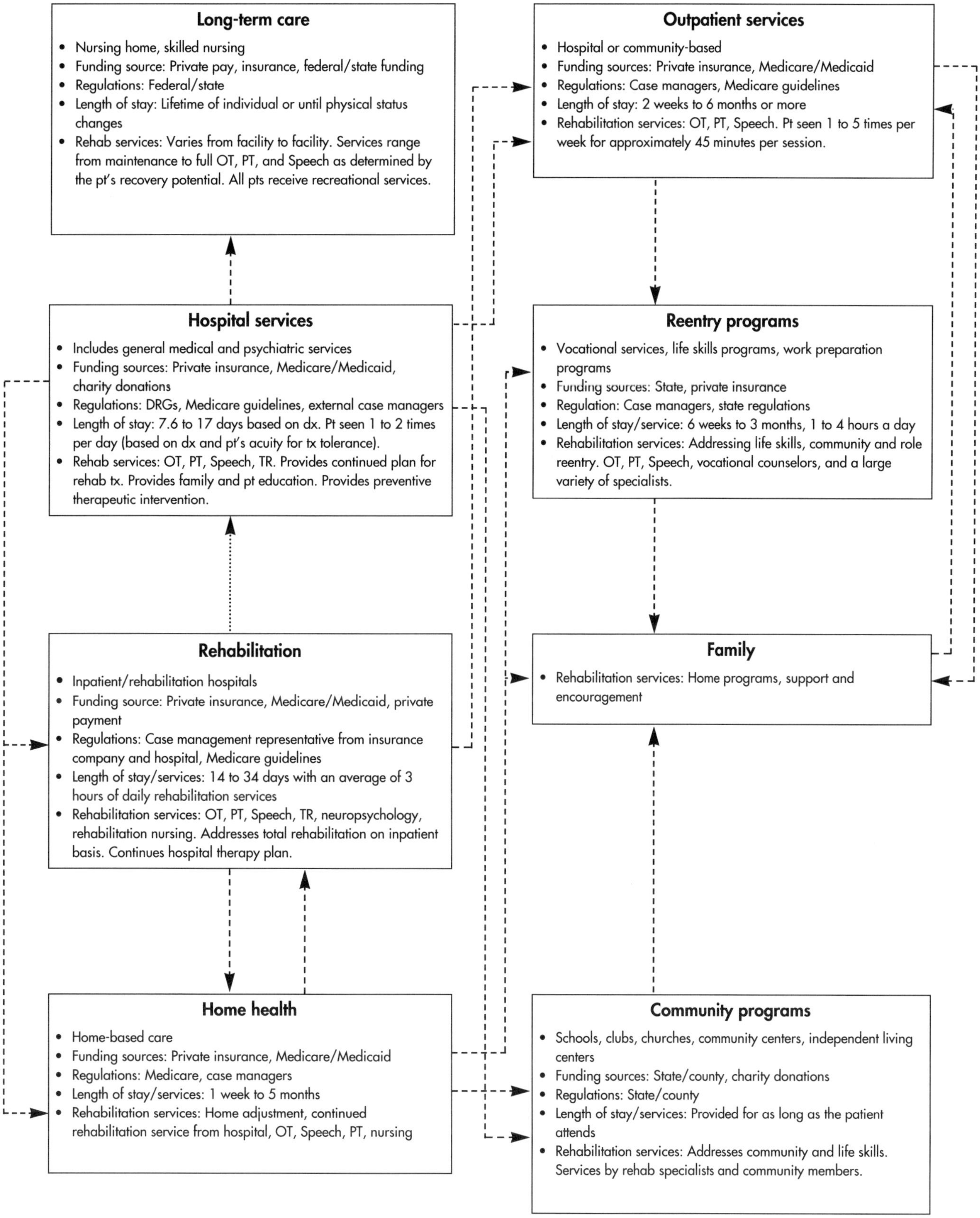

Figure 3.1. Health care continuum and common progression patterns in health care delivery. Adapted with permission from Baum, C. and Christiansen, C. *Occupational therapy: Overcoming human performance deficits,* Thorofare, NJ: Slack Incorporated.

type of therapy treatment from their family. A well-educated family and support system can continue to improve the patient's level of independence (see Figure 3.1).

Hospital Services

Hospital services include a large variety of medically based treatment. Most physical and psychiatric services begin in a hospital setting. While the majority of hospitals are considered to be non-profit organizations, they still need to consider financial reimbursement in order to maintain a staff and equipment. The common funding sources are private insurance, federal and state funding (i.e., Medicare and Medicaid), donations, and private payment by consumers.

Regulators that affect a patient's length of stay and the services that will be provided are the diagnosis related groups (DRGs), state and federal guidelines (i.e., Medicare and Medicaid), and case managers who represent private insurance companies.

Today the average length of the hospital stay ranges from 7.6 to 17 days, depending on the diagnosis. The most common rehabilitation services provided are occupational therapy, physical therapy, speech, and therapeutic recreation. Patients are seen 1 or 2 times per day, depending on their endurance. The primary focus of treatment is therapeutic intervention, preventative treatment techniques, family education, and a therapeutic plan that assists with discharge recommendations.

Long-Term Care

Long-term care includes nursing homes and skilled nursing facilities. The term *long-term care* is used frequently because of the stigma associated with nursing homes. They are frequently identified as a place to wait to die regardless of the services that are provided.

There is a new trend developing in the long-term care-institution. Many facilities are providing rehabilitation services to patients that focus on independent living skills within the facility. This method is intended to decrease the burden of care and/or facilitate the patient's transition back to his or her family and home.

The changes in long-term care evolved from the economic need to decrease the cost of care to the patient. It is important to know well in advance whether or not rehabilitation services will be available to patients being placed in long-term-care facilities in order to be able to adjust the treatment recommendations according to the patient's needs.

The funding sources for long-term care are generally the federal and state governments, insurance companies, and private payments. Regulations are instituted along state and federal guidelines. The length of stay can range from the lifetime of the individual to until there has been a physical or mental status change that may indicate a potential for functional independence. The primary rehabilitation service provided is physical therapy; occupational therapy and speech are also provided by physician referral.

Traditionally, the focus of therapeutic intervention is maintenance and recreational programming. Most long-term-care facilities contract for occupational therapy services. A consulting occupational therapist may provide services for 30 to 60 patients. Basic maintenance activities, such as passive range of motion and bed positioning, are generally done by the nursing staff after a consultation with physical therapy or occupational therapy.

Rehabilitation Services

A rehabilitation unit or hospital is designed to provide intensive rehabilitation services once the patient is medically stable. Rehabilitation services are provided by occupational therapy, physical therapy, speech, therapeutic recreation, and nursing. The average length of stay is 7 to 34 days, and most facilities offer 3 hours of direct therapy care per day.

Funding sources are generally private insurance, Medicare, and consumer payments. The rehabilitation process is regulated by federal guidelines and case managers representing private insurance companies. The focus of therapy is to provide an intense, total rehabilitation program that is also a continuation of the therapy process initiated in the acute care facility.

Outpatient Services

The current trend for rehabilitative care is to improve and expand outpatient services. This is viewed as a cost-effective method of delivering health care. The patient receives the benefit of rehabilitative care in a hospital or clinical setting while at home so the facilities do not incur the expense of 24-hour patient care.

Traditionally, most outpatient care was delivered through the hospital. Today, there are many different types of facilities that specialize in outpatient therapy. Hospitals have developed satellite facilities, physicians' offices provide therapy, and there is a growing number of clinics that are operated by therapists. Funding sources are generally private payment, private insurance, and Medicare. The current trend is for the system to be regulated by federal and state case managers.

The length of service varies greatly. A patient may be seen 1 to 5 times a week; the diagnosis and patient's status determine the duration of treatment.

Rehabilitation services also vary with the type of clinic. Physical therapy, occupational therapy, and speech therapy are the major disciplines involved with outpatient rehabilitation. For example, staffing for an outpatient hand clinic will usually include occupational therapists and physical therapists. Outpatient services for neurological disorders will typically include occupational therapy, physical therapy, and speech.

Home Health Care

Many individuals receive home health care services. A therapist will go to the person's home and provide treatment. The funding sources are private payment, private insurance, and Medicare. The system is regulated by Medicare guidelines and case managers. The length of service also varies, depending on the patient's need. Usually it ranges from 1 week to 3 months.

The patient is commonly seen 1 to 3 times per week. The primary focus of home health services is to assist with the patient's adjustment to functioning in the home. Services are provided by physical therapy, occupational therapy, speech therapy, and nursing. Frequently, the patient must be homebound to receive these services.

Reentry Programs

Reentry programs are designed to provide therapeutic intervention for the patient to learn life skills, and for community and life role reentry. The focus of these types of programs are return-to-work, transitional living, driver retraining and adaptation, technology center, head injury, and vocational services.

The programs are funded by state governments and private insurance. Regulation is provided by the state and case managers. The length of service is 6 weeks to 3 months. The programs are set up to provide service for 1 to 4 hours a day with each patient.

The programs include a large variety of disciplines. A partial list includes occupational therapy, physical therapy, speech therapy, neuropsychology, vocational counseling, and therapeutic recreation.

Community Programs

Many community-based programs provide various degrees of rehabilitation care. Schools, clubs, churches, community centers, and independent living centers provide a range of therapeutic and support services for individuals who need assistance. The funding sources for some of these programs are the state and county governments. These programs also depend heavily on charitable donations. Regulations are instituted by the state and county. The patients can participate in programs for as long as they are qualified to attend.

The staff includes some rehabilitation specialists, such as occupational therapists or physical therapists, but these programs are also supervised by members of the community. Many of these community programs provide family support and education. They can also be used as respite care resources.

In most situations, the occupational therapist is not responsible for making the entire discharge placement decision. Frequently, the occupational therapist has no control over these issues but can provide valuable recommendations that influence the discharge placement process. When discharge placement arrangements are determined, it is the therapist's responsibility to assist the patient with the transition by making recommendations and educating the patient, family members, and/or future facility.

For example, Thelma is an 84-year-old woman who suffered a stroke. She will be placed in a long-term-care facility. The occupational therapist providing her care in the current facility may make the following recommendations:

To the future facility:

- OT p.r.n. to monitor splint wearing schedule, w/c and bed positioning
- Splint wearing schedule: 2 hrs on/2 hrs off

To the patient:

- Provide information to Thelma about therapeutic activities that will be available to ease her transition.

To the family:

- Provide family education related to PROM and benefits of bed positioning and getting out of bed as Thelma tolerates. This will enable the family to be able to participate in her care if they desire, and they will be informed advocates for Thelma.

■ Practical Applications

Complete the exercises on pages 121–132. Evaluate the information provided and determine an appropriate occupational therapy recommendation for continued–therapy intervention.

Section 2

Home Program Development

A well-developed home program is a controlled, educational mechanism for patients and/or caregivers to continue a therapeutic therapy plan independently. It can also serve as a safe transition to encourage a patient to be reintroduced to life roles in the home and community.

Frequently, after a hospitalization or the rehabilitative process, the patient and family members are unclear about what the patient can do safely upon returning home. A home program should address concerns of the patient and family to ease this transition.

Home programs also provide intervention strategies that enhance therapeutic and medical recovery. For example, suppose a woman had a surgical procedure to replace the metacarpal (MC) joints in her hand. The initial home program provided by the occupational therapist would include an exercise plan and strategies to reduce scarring and edema.

Components of a home program should include an explanation of the purpose and goals of the exercises or recommendations, and written instructions that consider the patient's level of understanding. The therapist should also provide the patient with his or her name and business telephone number in case the patient has any questions once the program at home has been implemented.

An explanation of the purpose and goals of the home program should be reviewed with the patient and the primary caregiver. The explanation should be reviewed verbally, and the patient or caregiver should be allowed time during the occupational therapy session to practice the recommendations and ask questions. A brief explanation should also be included in the written directions to enable the patients or caregivers to review it when they get home.

This process may appear redundant; however, DiMatteo (1991) indicates that there are many factors that will interfere with the patient's ability to completely understand treatment recommendations. For example, many times health professionals communicate information in medical jargon or in terms that are unfamiliar to the patient. Other times, the patient may be so anxious during the therapeutic process that it can interfere with memorization and learning.

Sometimes people are reluctant to ask questions when they are provided with new information. They do not want to appear as if they are not intelligent enough to understand the process that is being explained.

Finally, the person's actual level of intelligence and the ability to relate to a new disability can affect the learning process. Providing a clear explanation, an opportunity to practice, and a brief written explanation can be effective in overcoming these communication barriers and will help ensure that the individual will follow through with the plan.

Providing written directions can be difficult; especially for those patients who have impaired reading ability. Pictures and diagrams may be the patient's only way of following the program. However, patients with perception deficits may find it difficult to follow diagrams. Therefore, providing an understandable home program may be as challenging to a therapist's creative ability as in preparing the treatment plan itself.

The therapist should provide his or her name, business telephone phone, and credentials with every home program. A patient may feel more comfortable calling the therapist than the physician if he or she is having complications or symptom changes. Also, patients or primary caregivers may have questions related to the program once they are at home (see Figure 3.2).

There are three major types of information that therapists often provide in home programs: energy conservation or protection, exercises, and suggestions for reintegrating the patient into his or her family role or activities. A program may include only one type of information or may have all three types. This depends on the diagnosis and the amount of information the therapist has available.

The Home Program

- Explanation of the purpose and goals of the exercises
- Written instructions
- Therapist's name and business phone number

Figure 3.2. Essential components of home programs

For instance, a therapist who works with orthopedic patients may provide a home program for a patient with a total hip replacement after seeing him or her 1 day. The home program will be different for a patient with a total hip replacement who has been seen for 2 weeks. There will be similarities in preparation and exercises; however, the therapist who has seen the patient for 2 weeks will be able to provide more complete information in relation to life role reintegration. ▲

■ Practical Applications

Complete the exercises on pages 133–134. Provide a written home program for each patient.

References

Christiansen, C., & Baum, C. (1991). *Occupational therapy: Overcoming human performance deficits*). Thorofare, NJ: Slack.

DiMatteo, M. R. (1991). *The psychology of health, illness, and medical care* (pp. 309–311). Pacific Grove, CA: Brooks/Cole.

■ Exercises 1:1

The following exercises list statements that are commonly found in patient records. Using the terms below, identify each statement as *subjective, objective, assessment,* or *plan* information. Briefly state the relevance of each to an occupational therapy evaluation. You are encouraged to use any occupational therapy references that are available.

Hint: To determine the information's relevance, imagine in each case that there are 2 different patients about whom nothing is known. Then a piece of information is presented about one of the patients. How would that information change your approach to the patient or family members in terms of evaluation or treatment?

S = Subjective
O = Objective
A = Assessment
P = Plan

■ Exercise 1:1—Record A

___P___1. Example: Pt to wear forearm cast and come in for follow-up appointment and x-ray in 5 weeks.

Relevance: The patient may need adaptive training for one-handed dressing, bathing, and ADL. Monitor and provide training for edema control and exercises for exposed joints to minimize complications that can occur secondary to decreased general use of upper extremity.

_______2. Pt is primarily limited by ↓ 'd endurance for activities.

Relevance:

_______3. Speech report states: Pt shows min limitations $\bar{c}$ expressive language skills.

Relevance:

_______4. Ox saturation levels are 80% at rest $\bar{c}$ room air.

Relevance:

_______5. Pt's father reports that his daughter is a straight "A" student, very popular and outgoing, and never drinks alcohol. Reliability of the father has not been established. The pt is in hospital after a car accident while intoxicated. Records show hx of alcohol-related incidents.

Relevance:

_______6. X-ray shows comminuted fx of the (R) tibia.

Relevance:

_______7. Pt non-weight bearing 6–8 weeks on (R) LE and follow-up x-ray in 4 weeks.

Relevance:

_______8. Physician report states: Pt shows good potential for intensive rehabilitation.

Relevance:

_______9. CT scan of brain indicates infarct of (R) parietal lobe.
Relevance:

_______10. Student to be trained c̄ adaptive computer for completing homework assignments.
Relevance:

_______11. A pt who has been in the hospital for 3 days states: "I had a nice visit c̄ my sister in New York yesterday; I just got back this morning."
Relevance:

_______12. Nursing reports the pt does not have any problems c̄ hand-to-mouth self-feeding.
Relevance:

_______13. Pt to be started on Macrodantin for 10 days and follow-up c̄ urine culture.
Relevance:

_______14. OT report from previous facility states: Pt's primary limitation is cognitive functioning which interferes c̄ ADL.
Relevance:

Answers on pages 135–136.

■ Exercise 1:1—Record B

__S__1. Example: Social Services report states: Pt appears independent c̄ all aspects of self-care.

Relevance: Provides information that can guide the evaluation process. A brief evaluation process for ADL is indicated.

_______2. Speech reports that the pt is not reliable for communication 2° to receptive aphasia disorder.

Relevance:

_______3. Pt states: "My birthday is June 15, 1990.'

Relevance:

_______4. Recommend providing ADL training 5x per week to ↑ pt level of independence.

Relevance:

_______5. Nsg reports the pt appears depressed.

Relevance:

_______6. OT report from previous facility states: Pt requires min (A) for bathing and dressing 2° to ↓'d endurance.

Relevance:

_______7. Social Services reports that the pt shows questionable reliability for significant life hx.

Relevance:

_______8. Pt to be d/c'd to her home c̄ her husband as the primary caregiver.

Relevance:

_______9. Initiate bowel and bladder training program.

Relevance:

_______10. PT report states: Pt shows poor potential for ambulation at this time.
Relevance:

_______11. PT reports: Pt is able to ambulate 35 ft $\bar{c}$ wheeled walker and SBA.
Relevance:

_______12. Pt states: "I hurt all over."
Relevance:

_______13. Physician report states: "Pt shows good comprehension of current limitations."
Relevance:

_______14. Pt states: "I want to be able to go home $\bar{c}$ my wife and use my arm again."
Relevance:

_______15. Strength at (R) UE shows: F+ at shoulder girdle, G at elbow flex/ext, G at wrist flex/ext, and shows 50# grip strength by OT report.
Relevance:

Answers on pages 137–138.

■ Exercises 1:2

Based on the information in each evaluation, indicate which areas would be appropriate to evaluate using the following four factors:

- Diagnosis
- Phase of recovery
- Facility that is serving the patient
- Other significant areas that are not related to the patient diagnosis (e.g., discharge plans, subjective reports, funding resources, past diagnoses, and other areas not related to the patient's current diagnosis).

Complete each set of worksheets and evaluation checklists, using any resource that is applicable and the information provided in the case scenario. The first patient evaluation has been completed as an example. This exercise is designed to provide an initial outline of areas to be evaluated. It is not meant to be exhaustive. If a therapist has developed an outline related to the factors listed above, and during the evaluation identifies a deficit area not on the outline, then the evaluation may be adjusted to include that area.

■ Exercise 1:2—Patient A (example)

The patient is in a rehabilitation clinic. His dx is CHI. His medical chart indicates that he is in a coma and medically stable. Prior to injury, he was living at home and going to school full time. The patient had no significant medical complications prior to injury. LOS is 3–4 months. The standard OT tx for the facility is 1 hr q.d.

A) Diagnosis: CHI

- Review of common complications c̄ CHI:
  Various levels of consciousness
  Cranial nerves susceptible to injury
  Possible coma c̄ a variety of duration lengths
  Local lesions involving one area of the brain; diffuse lesions involving several areas
- Secondary effects:
  Intracranial hypotension
  ↑ in intracranial pressure
  Cerebral edema
  Intracranial hemorrhage

Resource: Dow, P.W. (1989). Traumatic brain injuries. In C.A. Trombly (Ed.), *Occupational therapy for physical dysfunction* (3rd ed., pp. 484–487). Baltimore, MD: Williams & Wilkins.

B) Phase of recovery/facility that is serving pt:

Postacute because he is medically stable and in a rehabilitation clinic

C) Facility considerations:

LOS: 3–4 months
1 hr of tx per day

D) Other significant areas related to the pt's dx:

Functional level prior to current medical status

Review the following Evaluation Checklist.

Exercise 1:2

Category	Rating			Comments
	R	SR	N/A	
A. Independent Living/Daily Living Skills				
Physical Daily Living Skills				
Grooming and Hygiene			X	Task too complicated for pt's level of functioning
Feeding/Eating		X		Swallowing
Dressing			X	Task too complicated for pt's level of functioning
Functional Mobility				
Bed Mobility	X			Beginning of developmental process; able to test rolling responses and back response in rolling
W/C Mobility			X	Task too complicated for pt's level of functioning
Transfers			X	Task too complicated for pt's level of functioning
Functional Ambulation			X	Task too complicated for pt's level of functioning
Functional Communication	X			Possible eye blink or active movement communication
Object Manipulation	X			Response to item being put in hand; grasp reflex or higher
Psychological/Emotional Daily Living Skills				
Self-Concept/Self-Identity			X	
Situational Coping		X		Can be monitored by stress reactions. Does pt know what is being said and done?
Community Involvement			X	Task too complicated for pt's level of functioning
Work				
Homemaking			X	Task too complicated for pt's level of functioning
Child Care/Parenting			X	Same as above
Employment Preparation			X	Same as above
Play/Leisure			X	Same as above

Evaluation Checklist

Patient Name: Patient A

LEGEND: R—RELEVANT; SR—SOMEWHAT RELEVANT; N/A—NOT APPLICABLE

Category	Rating			Comments
	R	SR	N/A	
B. Sensorimotor Components				
Neuromuscular				
Reflex Integration	X			Types of reflex patterns seen can indicate level of damage and recovery
Range of Motion				
PROM	X			Evaluate muscle and joint intensity
AROM	X			Evaluate any type of controlled movement; additions indicate progress from coma state
A/AROM	X			Evaluate any type of controlled movement; additions indicate progress from coma state
Gross and Fine Coordination				
Muscle Control	X			Evaluate any type of controlled movement; additions indicate progress from coma state
Coordination		X		Can evaluate if patient shows muscle control
Dexterity		X		Can evaluate if patient shows muscle control
Strength and Endurance			X	
Sensory Integration	X			Determine if patient becomes overstimulated by various types of sensory stimulation
Sensory Awareness	X			Determine if patient responds to protopathic, proprioception, olfactory, vestibular, gustatory, visual, and/or auditory sensations
Visual-Spatial Awareness			X	
Body Integration				
Body Schema		X		Can evaluate if patient shows muscle control
Postural Balance	X			Responses to being in sitting or standing (tilt table) positions
(B) Motor Coordination			X	Task too difficult for patient's level of functioning
·Right-Left Discrimination			X	Same as above
Visual-Motor Integration			X	Same as above
Crossing Midline			X	

Evaluation Checklist continued

Patient Name: Patient A

LEGEND: R—RELEVANT; SR—SOMEWHAT RELEVANT; N/A—NOT APPLICABLE

Category	Rating			Comments
	R	SR	N/A	
Praxis		X		Can evaluate if patient shows muscle control
C. Cognitive Components				
Orientation		X		If pt is able to communicate
Conceptualization/Comprehension		X		Same as above
Concentration			X	
Attention Span		X		If pt is able to communicate
Memory		X		Same as above
Cognitive Integration				
Generalizing			X	Task too difficult for pt's level of functioning
Problem Solving			X	Same as above
Defining or Evaluating a Problem			X	Same as above
Organizing a Plan			X	Same as above
Implementing a Plan			X	Same as above
Evaluating a Decision			X	Same as above
D. Psychosocial Components				
Self-Management				
Self-Expression		X		Evaluate pt's ability to communicate pain, discomfort with eyes, muscle control, or reflex responses
Self-Control			X	Task too difficult for pt's level of functioning
Dyadic Interaction		X		Evaluate if pt is able to communicate
Group Interaction			X	
E. Therapeutic Adaptations				
Orthotics	X			Evaluate pt for hand splints, foot drop splints, other positioning devices
Prosthetics			X	
Assistive/Adaptive Equipment		X		Positioning equipment or communication system

Evaluation Checklist continued

Patient Name: Patient A

LEGEND: R—RELEVANT; SR—SOMEWHAT RELEVANT; N/A—NOT APPLICABLE

Category	Rating			Comments
	R	SR	N/A	
F. Prevention				
Energy Conservation			X	
Joint Protection/Body Mechanics	X			Joint positioning secondary to tone variations to prevent complications
Positioning	X			Bed, w/c, chair to prevent contractures and medical complications
Coordination of Daily Living Activities			X	Task too difficult for pt level of functioning

Evaluation Checklist continued

Patient Name: Patient A

LEGEND: R—RELEVANT; SR—SOMEWHAT RELEVANT; N/A—NOT APPLICABLE

Evaluation chart adapted from the *Reference Manual of the Official Documents of the American Occupational Therapy Association, Inc.* (pp. VIII.22–23) by The American Occupational Therapy Association, 1986, Rockville, MD: Author.

■ Exercise 1:2—Patient B

The pt is seen as an outpatient 3 x per wk. Her dx is a (R) UE flexor tendon repair. Surgery was 3 days ago and sutures are still in place. Physician indicates: Provide splint, no PROM for the next 2 weeks, and provide an AROM home program. The pt had no significant medical complications prior to injury. Pt will be scheduled for a follow-up appointment $\bar{c}$ the physician in 3 wks.

A) Diagnosis:

B) Phase of recovery:

C) Facility considerations:

D) Other significant areas:

Complete the following Evaluation Checklist. Answers on pages 139–142.

Category	Rating			Comments
	R	SR	N/A	
A. Independent Living/Daily Living Skills				
Physical Daily Living Skills				
Grooming and Hygiene				
Feeding/Eating				
Dressing				
Functional Mobility				
Bed Mobility				
W/C Mobility				
Transfers				
Functional Ambulation				
Functional Communication				
Object Manipulation				
Psychological/Emotional Daily Living Skills				
Self-Concept/Self-Identity				
Situational Coping				
Community Involvement				
Work				
Homemaking				
Child Care/Parenting				
Employment Preparation				
Play/Leisure				

Evaluation Checklist

Patient Name: Patient B

LEGEND: R—RELEVANT; SR—SOMEWHAT RELEVANT; N/A—NOT APPLICABLE

Category	Rating			Comments
	R	SR	N/A	
B. Sensorimotor Components				
Neuromuscular				
Reflex Integration				
Range of Motion				
PROM				
AROM				
A/AROM				
Gross and Fine Coordination				
Muscle Control				
Coordination				
Dexterity				
Strength and Endurance				
Sensory Integration				
Sensory Awareness				
Visual-Spatial Awareness				
Body Integration				
Body Schema				
Postural Balance				
(B) Motor Coordination				
Right-Left Discrimination				
Visual-Motor Integration				
Crossing Midline				
Praxis				
C. Cognitive Components				
Orientation				
Conceptualization/Comprehension				

Evaluation Checklist continued

Patient Name: Patient B

LEGEND: R—RELEVANT; SR—SOMEWHAT RELEVANT; N/A—NOT APPLICABLE

Category	Rating			Comments
	R	SR	N/A	
Concentration				
Attention Span				
Memory				
Cognitive Integration				
Generalizing				
Problem Solving				
Defining or Evaluating a Problem				
Organizing a Plan				
Implementing a Plan				
Evaluating a Decision				
D. Psychosocial Components				
Self-Management				
Self-Expression				
Self-Control				
Dyadic Interaction				
Group Interaction				
E. Therapeutic Adaptations				
Orthotics				
Prosthetics				
Assistive/Adaptive Equipment				
F. Prevention				
Energy Conservation				
Joint Protection/Body Mechanics				
Positioning				
Coordination of Daily Living Activities				

Evaluation Checklist continued

Patient Name: Patient B

LEGEND: R—RELEVANT; SR—SOMEWHAT RELEVANT; N/A—NOT APPLICABLE

Evaluation chart adapted from the *Reference Manual of the Official Documents of the American Occupational Therapy Association, Inc.* (pp. VIII.22–23) by The American Occupational Therapy Association, 1986, Rockville, MD: Author.

■ Exercise 1:2—Patient C

The pt is a 78 y/o F in an acute care hospital with a d/c date of 1 wk to her home. She lives alone. Her dx is Parkinson's disease. Her medications have been adjusted and she is beginning to show more freedom in her movements. Prior to the episode, her family reports she was getting very confused. The OT department's standard is to see the pt 1 hr q.d.

A) Diagnosis:

B) Phase of recovery:

C) Facility considerations:

D) Other significant areas:

Complete the following Evaluation Checklist. Answers on pages 143–146.

Category	Rating			Comments
	R	SR	N/A	
A. Independent Living/Daily Living Skills				
Physical Daily Living Skills				
Grooming and Hygiene				
Feeding/Eating				
Dressing				
Functional Mobility				
Bed Mobility				
W/C Mobility				
Transfers				
Functional Ambulation				
Functional Communication				
Object Manipulation				
Psychological/Emotional Daily Living Skills				
Self-Concept/Self-Identity				
Situational Coping				
Community Involvement				
Work				
Homemaking				
Child Care/Parenting				
Employment Preparation				
Play/Leisure				

Evaluation Checklist

Patient Name: Patient C

LEGEND: R—RELEVANT; SR—SOMEWHAT RELEVANT; N/A—NOT APPLICABLE

Category	Rating			Comments
	R	SR	N/A	
B. Sensorimotor Components				
Neuromuscular				
Reflex Integration				
Range of Motion				
PROM				
AROM				
A/AROM				
Gross and Fine Coordination				
Muscle Control				
Coordination				
Dexterity				
Strength and Endurance				
Sensory Integration				
Sensory Awareness				
Visual-Spatial Awareness				
Body Integration				
Body Schema				
Postural Balance				
(B) Motor Coordination				
Right-Left Discrimination				
Visual-Motor Integration				
Crossing Midline				
Praxis				
C. Cognitive Components				
Orientation				
Conceptualization/Comprehension				

Evaluation Checklist continued

Patient Name: Patient C

LEGEND: R—RELEVANT; SR—SOMEWHAT RELEVANT; N/A—NOT APPLICABLE

Category	Rating			Comments
	R	SR	N/A	
Concentration				
Attention Span				
Memory				
Cognitive Integration				
Generalizing				
Problem Solving				
Defining or Evaluating a Problem				
Organizing a Plan				
Implementing a Plan				
Evaluating a Decision				
D. Psychosocial Components				
Self-Management				
Self-Expression				
Self-Control				
Dyadic Interaction				
Group Interaction				
E. Therapeutic Adaptations				
Orthotics				
Prosthetics				
Assistive/Adaptive Equipment				
F. Prevention				
Energy Conservation				
Joint Protection/Body Mechanics				
Positioning				
Coordination of Daily Living Activities				

Evaluation Checklist continued

Patient Name: Patient C

LEGEND: R—RELEVANT; SR—SOMEWHAT RELEVANT; N/A—NOT APPLICABLE

Evaluation chart adapted from the *Reference Manual of the Official Documents of the American Occupational Therapy Association, Inc.* (pp. VIII.22–23) by The American Occupational Therapy Association, 1986, Rockville, MD: Author.

■ Exercise 1:2 —Patient D

The pt is a 6 y/o girl with spina bifida. The therapy schedule is 1x per week throughout the year in the school she is attending as a mainstreamed student. There are no other medical complications identified.

A) Diagnosis:

B) Phase of recovery:

C) Facility considerations:

D) Other significant areas:

Complete the following Evaluation Checklist. Answers on pages 147–151.

Category	Rating			Comments
	R	SR	N/A	
A. Independent Living/Daily Living Skills				
Physical Daily Living Skills				
Grooming and Hygiene				
Feeding/Eating				
Dressing				
Functional Mobility				
Bed Mobility				
W/C Mobility				
Transfers				
Functional Ambulation				
Functional Communication				
Object Manipulation				
Psychological/Emotional Daily Living Skills				
Self-Concept/Self-Identity				
Situational Coping				
Community Involvement				
Work				
Homemaking				
Child Care/Parenting				
Employment Preparation				
Play/Leisure				

Evaluation Checklist

Patient Name: Patient D

LEGEND: R—RELEVANT; SR—SOMEWHAT RELEVANT; N/A—NOT APPLICABLE

Category	Rating			Comments
	R	SR	N/A	
B. Sensorimotor Components				
Neuromuscular				
Reflex Integration				
Range of Motion				
PROM				
AROM				
A/AROM				
Gross and Fine Coordination				
Muscle Control				
Coordination				
Dexterity				
Strength and Endurance				
Sensory Integration				
Sensory Awareness				
Visual-Spatial Awareness				
Body Integration				
Body Schema				
Postural Balance				
(B) Motor Coordination				
Right-Left Discrimination				
Visual-Motor Integration				
Crossing Midline				
Praxis				
C. Cognitive Components				
Orientation				
Conceptualization/Comprehension				

Evaluation Checklist continued

Patient Name: Patient D

LEGEND: R—RELEVANT; SR—SOMEWHAT RELEVANT; N/A—NOT APPLICABLE

Category	Rating			Comments
	R	SR	N/A	
Concentration				
Attention Span				
Memory				
Cognitive Integration				
Generalizing				
Problem Solving				
Defining or Evaluating a Problem				
Organizing a Plan				
Implementing a Plan				
Evaluating a Decision				
D. Psychosocial Components				
Self-Management				
Self-Expression				
Self-Control				
Dyadic Interaction				
Group Interaction				
E. Therapeutic Adaptations				
Orthotics				
Prosthetics				
Assistive/Adaptive Equipment				
F. Prevention				
Energy Conservation				
Joint Protection/Body Mechanics				
Positioning				
Coordination of Daily Living Activities				

Evaluation Checklist continued

Patient Name: Patient D

LEGEND: R—RELEVANT; SR—SOMEWHAT RELEVANT; N/A—NOT APPLICABLE

Evaluation chart adapted from the *Reference Manual of the Official Documents of the American Occupational Therapy Association, Inc.* (pp. VIII.22–23) by The American Occupational Therapy Association, 1986, Rockville, MD: Author.

■ Exercise 1:2—Patient E

The pt has a dx of THR with a hx of severe RA (posterior approach). Her therapy is scheduled 30 minutes q.d. for 2 weeks in an acute care hospital. She lives in a nursing home. Her discharge plan is to return to the nursing home. The pt has multiple joint deformities, including min functioning shoulder joints and nonfunctioning fingers.

A) Diagnosis:

B) Phase of recovery:

C) Facility considerations:

D) Other significant areas:

Complete the following Evaluation Checklist. Answers on pages 152–155.

Category	Rating			Comments
	R	SR	N/A	
A. Independent Living/Daily Living Skills				
Physical Daily Living Skills:				
Grooming and Hygiene				
Feeding/Eating				
Dressing				
Functional Mobility				
Bed Mobility				
W/C Mobility				
Transfers				
Functional Ambulation				
Functional Communication				
Object Manipulation				
Psychological/Emotional Daily Living Skills				
Self-Concept/Self-Identity				
Situational Coping				
Community Involvement				
Work				
Homemaking				
Child Care/Parenting				
Employment Preparation				
Play/Leisure				

Evaluation Checklist

Patient Name: Patient E

LEGEND: R—RELEVANT; SR—SOMEWHAT RELEVANT; N/A—NOT APPLICABLE

Category	Rating			Comments
	R	SR	N/A	
B. Sensorimotor Components				
Neuromuscular				
Reflex Integration				
Range of Motion				
PROM				
AROM				
A/AROM				
Gross and Fine Coordination				
Muscle Control				
Coordination				
Dexterity				
Strength and Endurance				
Sensory Integration				
Sensory Awareness				
Visual-Spatial Awareness				
Body Integration				
Body Schema				
Postural Balance				
(B) Motor Coordination				
Right-Left Discrimination				
Visual-Motor Integration				
Crossing Midline				
Praxis				
C. Cognitive Components				
Orientation				
Conceptualization/Comprehension				

Evaluation Checklist continued

Patient Name: Patient E

LEGEND: R—RELEVANT; SR—SOMEWHAT RELEVANT; N/A—NOT APPLICABLE

Category	Rating			Comments
	R	SR	N/A	
Concentration				
Attention Span				
Memory				
Cognitive Integration				
Generalizing				
Problem Solving				
Defining or Evaluating a Problem				
Organizing a Plan				
Implementing a Plan				
Evaluating a Decision				
D. Psychosocial Components				
Self-Management				
Self-Expression				
Self-Control				
Dyadic Interaction				
Group Interaction				
E. Therapeutic Adaptations				
Orthotics				
Prosthetics				
Assistive/Adaptive Equipment				
F. Prevention				
Energy Conservation				
Joint Protection/Body Mechanics				
Positioning				
Coordination of Daily Living Activities				

Evaluation Checklist continued

Patient Name: Patient E

LEGEND: R—RELEVANT; SR—SOMEWHAT RELEVANT; N/A—NOT APPLICABLE

Evaluation chart adapted from the *Reference Manual of the Official Documents of the American Occupational Therapy Association, Inc.* (pp. VIII.22–23) by The American Occupational Therapy Association, 1986, Rockville, MD: Author.

■ Exercise 1:2—Patient F

The pt has a dx of CVA s/p 3 days. The CT scan showed an occlusion of the internal carotid artery. Pt is currently in the ICU. Prior to this injury, pt was retired and lived with his wife independently. Other medical complications include MI s/p 6 months and IDDM. He will be seen in the ICU, followed to the acute care floor, and transferred to a rehab unit.

A) Diagnosis:

B) Phase of recovery:

C) Facility considerations:

D) Other significant areas:

Complete the following Evaluation Checklist. Answers on pages 156–159.

Category	Rating			Comments
	R	SR	N/A	
A. Independent Living/Daily Living Skills				
Physical Daily Living Skills				
Grooming and Hygiene				
Feeding/Eating				
Dressing				
Functional Mobility				
Bed Mobility				
W/C Mobility				
Transfers				
Functional Ambulation				
Functional Communication				
Object Manipulation				
Psychological/Emotional Daily Living Skills				
Self-Concept/Self-Identity				
Situational Coping				
Community Involvement				
Work				
Homemaking				
Child Care/Parenting				
Employment Preparation				
Play/Leisure				

Evaluation Checklist

Patient Name: Patient F

LEGEND: R—RELEVANT; SR—SOMEWHAT RELEVANT; N/A—NOT APPLICABLE

Category	Rating R	Rating SR	Rating N/A	Comments
B. Sensorimotor Components				
Neuromuscular				
Reflex Integration				
Range of Motion				
PROM				
AROM				
A/AROM				
Gross and Fine Coordination				
Muscle Control				
Coordination				
Dexterity				
Strength and Endurance				
Sensory Integration				
Sensory Awareness				
Visual-Spatial Awareness				
Body Integration				
Body Schema				
Postural Balance				
(B) Motor Coordination				
Right-Left Discrimination				
Visual-Motor Integration				
Crossing Midline				
Praxis				
C. Cognitive Components				
Orientation				
Conceptualization/Comprehension				

Evaluation Checklist continued

Patient Name: Patient F

LEGEND: R—RELEVANT; SR—SOMEWHAT RELEVANT; N/A—NOT APPLICABLE

Category	Rating			Comments
	R	SR	N/A	
Concentration				
Attention Span				
Memory				
Cognitive Integration				
Generalizing				
Problem Solving				
Defining or Evaluating a Problem				
Organizing a Plan				
Implementing a Plan				
Evaluating a Decision				
D. Psychosocial Components				
Self-Management				
Self-Expression				
Self-Control				
Dyadic Interaction				
Group Interaction				
E. Therapeutic Adaptations				
Orthotics				
Prosthetics				
Assistive/Adaptive Equipment				
F. Prevention				
Energy Conservation				
Joint Protection/Body Mechanics				
Positioning				
Coordination of Daily Living Activities				

Evaluation Checklist continued

Patient Name: Patient F

LEGEND: R—RELEVANT; SR—SOMEWHAT RELEVANT; N/A—NOT APPLICABLE

Evaluation chart adapted from the *Reference Manual of the Official Documents of the American Occupational Therapy Association, Inc.* (pp. VIII.22–23) by The American Occupational Therapy Association, 1986, Rockville, MD: Author.

■ Exercises 1:3

Read the following evaluations carefully. Answer the questions that follow each one. You are encouraged to use any occupational therapy references that are available.

Exercise 1:3a—Margaret

Margaret is a 58 y/o F referred to occupational therapy.

Referral reads:

- Dx: hip fx
- Please evaluate and provide tx.

Medical chart information:

- THR (L), s/p 2 days surgery
- Hypertension
- DJD, mild throughout body
- Pt d/c plan 1 week to home
- (B) WBAT
- Pt fell off curb getting into car when she was leaving a restaurant.
- Margaret enjoys cooking, works as a receptionist, and is very active in church functions.

Medications

- Percocet N100 p.r.n.
- ASA
- Heparin

The facility uses the following guidelines for THR precautions:

- Do not flex hips past 90°
- No internal or external rotation of hip
- No adduction of hips past neutral

Exercise 1:3a

A) List the possible reasons for Margaret's prescribed medications and the potential side effects.

B) When talking with Margaret during her interview, she appears to be oriented, alert, and a reliable source for information. What type of information would be important to obtain during the interview?

C) What physical status information is needed to evaluate the patient, and why?

D) What cognitive status information is needed to evaluate the patient, and why?

E) Based on what is known about the patient evaluation and therapy process, what information is needed from the physical therapist before household mobility training is started?

F) Identify the areas of therapy that would need to be addressed with Margaret to help her return home safely.

Answers on page 160.

■ Exercise 1:3b—Beulah

Beulah is a 79 y/o F. She is placed in a rehabilitation unit for physical and occupational therapy services.

Referral reads:

- Dx: (R) hip fx c̄ THR
- Evaluate and treat.

Medical chart information:

- Hx of Parkinson's disease
- UTI
- THR (R), 2 days s/p
- (B) WBAT
- Patient to be poseyed at all times.
- Patient lives with her daughter Carol.

Medications:

- Parlodel
- Macrodantin
- Tylenol® #3 p.r.n.
- Guidelines for total hip precautions as indicated on Exercise 1:3a—Margaret.

As you approach Beulah, she is in a wheelchair with a waist posey and she is carrying a towel. She is talking very quietly to herself. The initial interview is as follows:

Thelma (Therapist): Hi, Beulah, my name is Thelma. I am an occupational therapist. Your doctor asked me to see you to help you get back on your feet.

Beulah: Nice to meet you, Thelma. Thanks for coming over. Would you like something to eat?

Thelma: No, thank you. Beulah, do you know where you are?

Beulah: Why, yes. I am at home with my mother and father. This is my baby, Tami. Isn't she sweet?

Thelma: Beulah, you are in the hospital right now. Do you live alone?

Beulah: Yes, I've lived alone all my life. My good plates are gone. Someone must have stolen them. (Beulah begins to cry.)

Thelma: I am sure your plates are with your daughter Carol. (Beulah becomes more comfortable.)

Thelma gets some bright-colored pegs and a bucket and puts them on a table in front of Beulah.

Thelma: Can you put these pegs in this bucket for me, please?

Beulah: Sure I can. (Beulah tries to reach up for the pegs; her movements are slow and appear rigid. She is unable to complete putting the pegs in the bucket without physical and verbal cues.)

Exercise 1:3b

A) List possible reasons for Beulah's medications and what side effects you would have to consider.

B) What is wrong with Beulah's cognitive status, and how could you word it in an initial note?

C) What are two possible reasons for Beulah's cognitive status?

D) What other hospital service could you contact to get a history and living situation on Beulah, and what kind of information do you need?

E) Assuming Beulah's mental status is a permanent condition, is she an appropriate candidate for a rehabilitation setting? If she is, what areas would you concentrate on for further evaluation?

Answers on page 161.

■ Exercise 1:3c—Tom

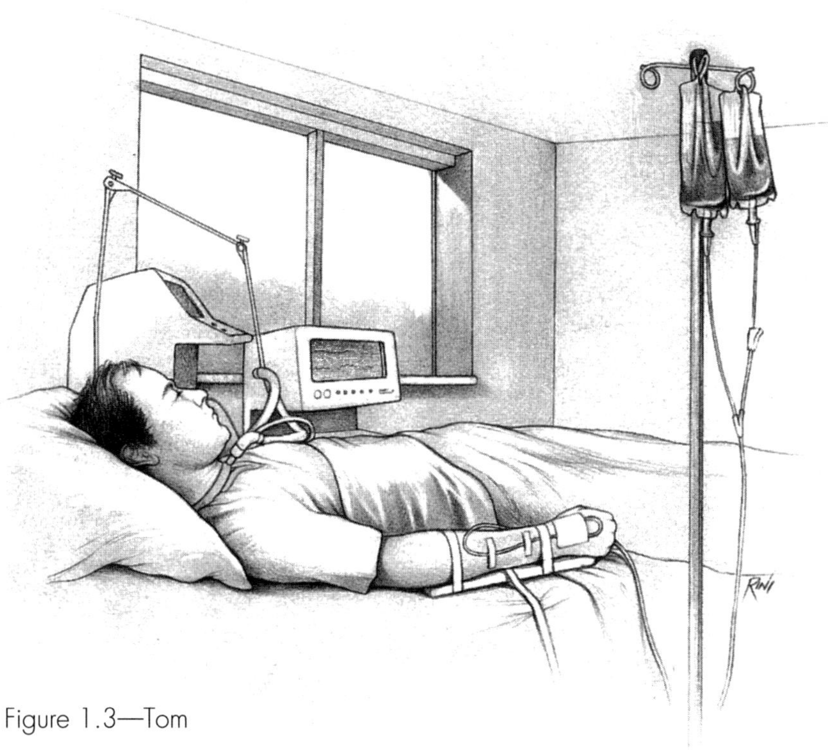

Figure 1.3—Tom

Tom is an 82 y/o M in an ICU.

Referral reads:

- Dx: L CVA
- Evaluate and treat.

Medical chart information:

- R parietal CVA s/p 2 days
- DM
- MI s/p 2 months
- Patient lives with wife and required her assistance for ADL prior to admit.

Medications:

- Heparin
- Procardia
- Humulin insulin NPH (neutral protamine hagedorn–long-acting)

When you approach Tom, he is in bed supine with an IV in his right arm, a urinary catheter, and three leads from an ECG monitor on his chest for tracking his heart condition. He appears very tired and is slow to respond to your questions. Treatment should be kept very short because of his medical condition.

Exercise 1:3c

A) List possible reasons for Tom's medications and what side effects you would have to consider.

B) How would you evaluate his mental status?

C) What would you evaluate in his right UE and why?

D) What would you evaluate in his left UE and why?

E) How could you do a simple test for visual neglect?

F) Tom's left arm is flaccid, and he appears unable to move it. How can you determine if he has any movement in his arm?

Answers on page 162.

■ Exercise 1:3d—Ed

Ed is a 56 y/o M who was admitted to the rehabilitation unit.

Referral reads:

- Dx: (L) CVA
- Evaluate and treat.

Medical chart information:

- (L) parietal lobe infarct
- Hypertension

Medications:

- Coumadin
- Verapamil hydrochloride

Ed is a large, well-built man. He is seated in a wheelchair and looking to his extreme left. The initial interview is as follows:

Larry (Therapist): Hi, Ed. My name is Larry. I am an occupational therapist and our doctor asked me to see you. (Larry continues to explain the role of OT. Ed continues to look to his left and says nothing.)

Larry: Ed, can you please look at me?

(Ed follows Larry's voice to the right to look at Larry for a couple of seconds and then turns his head back to the left.)

Larry: Do you live alone?

Ed: Ahhhhhhh Ahhhhhhh Ah Ah

Larry: Okay, Ed, try this. Just shake your head "yes" or "no." Do you live alone?

(Ed shakes his head "yes.")

Larry: Are you a man?

(Ed shakes his head "no.")

Exercise 1:3d

A) List the possible reasons for Ed's medications and the side effects you would look for.

B) What could be the possible reasons for Ed being unable to look at Larry, and how would you further evaluate the severity of his problem?

C) Assuming Ed has no other therapy referrals, what other rehabilitation services would you recommend based on the interview? Why?

D) From what service could you get personal information about Ed, and what kinds of things would you need to know?

E) What areas would you evaluate next? How?

Answers on page 163.

■ Exercise 1:3e—Warren

Warren is a 68 y/o M on a rehabilitation unit to receive his prosthesis and gait training.

Referral reads:

- Eval/tx for ADL status.

Medical chart information:

- (R) BKA s/p 1 week
- IDDM
- Cardiac arrhythmia
- Questionable hx of ETOH abuse

Medications:

- Humulin insulin NPH
- Inderal
- Tylenol® #3 p.r.n.

In the interview, Warren indicates he is a retired high school coach. He swam every day up until 2 weeks before surgery, and he enjoys playing golf. Warren is complaining of pain in his (R) foot while he is sitting in his chair and says it is worse at night while he is sleeping.

Exercise 1:3e

A) List the possible reasons for Warren's medications and the side effects you will have to consider.

B) What is wrong with Warren's right foot? What type of therapy approaches can you provide to try to decrease Warren's discomfort?

C) What areas would you evaluate with Warren before he receives his prosthesis, and why?

D) Warren has received his prosthesis, and physical therapy reports that he is walking fairly well with a walker. What areas would you address to assist his progress to a cane and what activities would you provide as therapy? After each therapy session, what would you need to do with Warren to make sure his prosthesis is a correct fit?

E) Would you need to address transfers and mobility without the prosthesis? Why or why not?

F) Identify three areas of focus for Warren's therapy plan.

Answers on pages 164–165.

■ Exercise 1:3f—Sara

Sara is a 23 y/o F currently in an acute care facility with the possibility of going to a rehabilitation unit.

Referral reads:

- Dx: (L) UE below–elbow amputee
- Eval the potential for UE prosthesis.

Medical chart information:

- (L) UE below–elbow amputee s/p 1 week.
- No other significant medical hx.

Sara was involved in a car accident. She enjoys horseback riding, reading, and playing various sports. She works as a data processor. She is currently taking various courses at the community college, with no major declared.

Exercise 1:3f

A) What areas would you evaluate to help make your recommendation for prosthesis training?

B) What other service could you contact to determine the financial and insurance information you need to help determine your recommendations? What information do you need to know?

C) Are there any areas you can effectively treat now? If so, list them and explain how you would approach the physician for a referral for treatment until Sara's discharge plans are final.

Answers on page 166.

■ Exercise 1:3g—Phillip

Phillip is a 9 y/o M in a rehabilitation unit. He has received referrals for occupational therapy, physical therapy, speech and language pathology, social services, and recreational therapy, as well as the referral listed below.

Referral reads:

- Dx: CHI
- Eval and tx; focus on positioning and current functional status; provide w/c to get patient OOB

Medical chart information:

- CHI via MVA s/p 2 months
- Extubation of trach tube s/p 2 weeks
- Colostomy s/p 6 weeks

X-ray reports:

- (R) frontal and parietal lobe damage
- No fx sites noted
- Diffuse trauma throughout brain

Medications:

- Dilantin
- Bactrim

Phillip was a passenger in an MVA. Prior to the accident, he attended 4th grade public school. He has an average to high grade point average. He enjoys soccer, Teenage Mutant Ninja Turtles, and video games.

Phillip is unable to speak. He has no reliable communication system. He cries every time he is moved. To make the evaluation sessions less stressful for him, it was mutually decided by the treatment team to combine the occupational therapy evaluation with the other disciplines. Phillip is being seen bedside and he is completely flaccid.

Exercise 1:3g

A) What areas do you need to evaluate to provide a temporary wheelchair? (Hint: Consider the pt head to toe.)

B) Is there any information you can get from nursing to assist you in evaluating wheelchair equipment needs?

C) What areas will you evaluate when you are working with physical therapy?

D) What areas will you evaluate when you are working with speech and language pathology?

Answers on page 167.

■ Exercise 1:3h—Nancy

Nancy is a 32 y/o F. She is an outpatient referred to your clinic.

Referral reads:

- Dx: RA
- Eval for baseline information and provide education for arthritis care.

Medical chart information:

- RA, onset 1 year ago
- Nancy is a homemaker with two children, 7 and 4 years old. Her primary complaint is joint pain currently confined to her hands.

Medications:

- Nonsteroidal antiinflamatory (NSAID)
- Prednisone injection to (L) shoulder 2 days ago

Exercise 1:3h

A) List the possible reasons for Nancy's medication and what precautions you may need to take.

B) What areas would you evaluate and document? Why?

C) During the evaluation you discover Nancy is developing ulnar deviation in both hands. Is there anything you can do?

D) How would you approach the doctor with this subject? How would you explain the rationale for your recommended therapy to the doctor?

Answers on page 168.

■ Exercise 1:3i—Timothy

Timothy is a 22 y/o M in a long-term rehabilitation facility. He has not been out of bed since his injury.

Referral reads:

- Dx: spinal cord injury
- Eval and tx.

Medical chart information:

- C-5–C-6 spinal cord injury incomplete.

Medications:

- Colace
- Metamucil/Dulcolax
- Valium

Tim was involved in a diving accident 4 weeks ago. There was suspected ETOH use at the time of injury. Tim works as a car mechanic. He has a high school education and no prior interest in college. Tim enjoys motorcycles and "hanging out" with his friends.

Exercise 1:3i

A) List the possible reasons for Tim's medications and what precautions you would need to keep in mind.

B) What areas would you need to evaluate to develop your therapy plan? Why?

C) Would it be appropriate to work with another discipline for any areas of your evaluation? If so, what areas and which discipline(s) would you consult or work with?

D) What precautions would you need to take before you evaluate Tim's gross motor skills? Why?

Answers on pages 169–170.

■ Exercise 1:3j—Mary

Mary is a 42 y/o F in an acute care hospital.

Referral reads:

- Dx: aneurysm
- Eval and tx.

Medical chart information:

- Aneurysm burst s/p 1 week; patient underwent clipping for 2 aneurysms s/p 1 week. Location involved cerebellum and (L) temporal lobe.
- CT of head indicates min edema. Lesions in (L) temporal lobe and cerebellum.

Mary was preparing dinner for her family. She indicated she had a headache earlier that evening to her husband. She told her husband she was feeling sick to her stomach and went to lay down. Her husband went to check on her about 45 minutes later and was unable to wake her. She was taken to the hospital and underwent evacuation for the hemorrhage, followed by a CT of the head. The following day, she underwent surgery for clipping of another aneurysm.

Medications:

- Nimodipine for 21 days
- Heparin

Mary is in a regular w/c. She is alert and has her hands lying in her lap. You explain that you are an occupational therapist and why she is here to see you. You ask Mary how she is feeling today and she doesn't reply. You then ask her to raise her arms up in the air. Mary looks away from you and grasps her hands together in her lap.

Exercise 1:3j

A) List the possible reasons for Mary's medications and the side effects that could occur.

B) Considering the injury sites of the brain, what are the possible reasons for Mary's responses to your requests?

C) How will you determine more accurately what Mary's problems are for the evaluation?

D) List the other areas you would evaluate and why.

Answers on pages 171–172.

■ Exercises 2:1

Read all the patient information that is provided in each exercise. Complete Question D of each evaluation. You are encouraged to use any occupational therapy references that are available.

■ Exercise 2:1a—Anne (example)

A) Where is Anne now?

Anne is an 87 y/o F with a dx of multiple fractures secondary to a fall. She has a fx (R) tibia and a fx (R) radius. Currently, she is in full leg and full arm casts. Anne has been living in a nursing home for the past 5 years. Her medical hx includes dementia and osteoporosis. Anne's precautions are non-weight bearing on (R) LE or (R) UE.

B) What is Anne's current status?

UE status: (R)UE PROM at shoulder WFL, strength not formally tested 2° to cast and the patient's poor direction following. Fingers and thumb show moderate edema. Color of fingers and nail beds pink, (L) UE AROM WFL; strength appears about fair throughout, but not formally tested. Coordination is moderately impaired.

Cog status: Pt not oriented to time or place. She is confused and has difficulty following simple directions. She is able to complete simple automatic responses and tasks. The patient occasionally cries in tx, apparently 2° to confusion.

Transfers: Pt requires max (A) to transfer w/c ↔ mat. She is unable to monitor the current nonweight bearing status on her (R) LE.

Gross motor skills: Rolling (R) and (L) requires mod (A); sit ↔ supine requires max (A). Pt appears fearful of moving.

Self-care: Pt dependent for donning/doffing sweater. She requires min (A) to feed self with nondominant hand. Other bathing & dressing dependent.

C) What are Anne's goals?

Anne will be returning to the nursing home. Before the fall, Anne was able to feed herself, get in and out of bed $\bar{c}$ SBA, and perform bed mobility independently.

D) How can Anne reach these goals?

1. Identify Anne's strengths and weaknesses

Strengths:

- (L) UE AROM and strength are functional.
- Discharge placement is defined.
- (L) UE is functional.

Weaknesses:

- Cognitive status (confusion and fear)
- ↓'d mobility (bed and transfers)
- ↓'d self-feeding

2. Identify the major skills Anne will need to enable her to reach her desired destination. (List long-range goals).

- ↑ transfer ability; ↓ fear; and ↑safety
- ↑ self-feeding skills.
- ↑ bed mobility skills.

All these skills will assist the caregivers in caring for Anne.

3. What specific skills will you need to address in order to work toward the major skills listed above? Why? (List short-term goals.)

- Weight bearing on (L) LE only to maintain circulation in order to work toward transferring using (L) LE only.
- Trunk rotation activities in chair to ↓ fear of movement.
- Coordination activities $\bar{c}$ (L) UE to work toward self-feeding.

4. Identify two specific activities per area addressed in Section 3 above.

- Have Anne stand at counter $\bar{c}$ your foot under her (L) LE and have her separate silverware.
- Practice transfers.
- Have Anne sit in a regular chair at a table and help you fold towels $\bar{c}$ 1 hand.
- Have Anne sit EOM and pick up pegs on her (L) side (using her right hand) and throw them away in a trash can on her (R) side.
- Practice self-feeding; start $\bar{c}$ finger foods.
- Play cards $\bar{c}$ a card holder; have Anne put the cards in a holder.

■ Exercise 2:1b—Carol

A) Where is Carol now?

Carol is a 28 y/o F with a dx of uncontrolled DM. She is legally blind in both eyes. She had a (R) BKA 6 months prior to current admission. She is now admitted because of gangrene in (L) foot and ankle. She has been admitted to receive whirlpool tx to the (L) LE, IV antibiotic tx, and possible amputation of (L) ankle/foot if infection remains uncontrollable. General prognosis to save the (L) LE is poor.

B) What is Carol's current status?

Subjective information: Carol reports she feels she is getting more dependent on her mother every day, and she doesn't like it.

Transfers: Pt indep c̄ functional transfers using crutches and weight bearing on (L) LE. Tub transfers indep c̄ crutches and tub transfer bench.

Gross motor mobility: Independent rolling (R) and (L). She requires min (A) sit↔supine.

Equipment: Pt has transfer tub bench, crutches, and exercise equipment for UE and LE activities.

UE functioning: Pt's UEs are WFL (B) for AROM; strength is good– (B). No sign of edema or skin tears noted. UE sensation stereognosis generally intact; sharp/dull and temperature impaired (B). Proprioception intact (B). Pt's gross motor coordination is WFL (B). Fine motor coordination is impaired (B) which appears 2° to ↓'d sensation in finger tip region.

Self-care skills: Pt requires mod (A) for dressing 2° to poor ability to orient clothes and requires (A) for standing during LE dressing. Bathing skills independent. Grooming skills require set-up.

C) What are Carol's goals?

Carol was an RN and living in her own apartment until 1 year ago. She moved in c̄ her mother when her health deteriorated and she had to quit work. She will be returning home c̄ her mother. Both Carol and her mother realize that Carol's care is becoming more difficult as time passes. Carol feels very guilty that she is becoming totally dependent on her mother. Carol's primary concern is that she doesn't want her mother to have to lift her. Both Carol and her mother feel their relationship has changed, and they don't have anything they can enjoy and do together any more.

Exercise 2:1b

D) How can Carol reach her goals?

1. Identify Carol's strengths and weaknesses.

2. Identify the major skills Carol will need to enable her to reach her desired destination. (List long-range goals.)

3. What specific skills will you need to address in order to work toward the major skills listed above? Why? (List short-term goals.)

4. Identify two specific activities per area addressed in Section 3 above.

Answers on page 173.

■ Exercise 2:1c—Kevin

A) Where is Kevin now?

Kevin is a 22 y/o c̄ dx of spinal cord injury—incomplete T-6. Kevin's hx includes falling off the roof of his family's home while cleaning gutters 1 year ago. He progressed from an acute care rehab program 4 months ago and went home c̄ his family. Since Kevin has been home, he has been mostly staying in his house and yard. When he goes out, his father helps him c̄ his equipment and car transfers.

B) What is Kevin's current status?

UE status: AROM is WFL. Strength is normal or above for his age.

Cognitive status: Pt cog status intact for following complex directions. Pt shows good judgment and safety awareness.

Transfers: Bed and toilet transfers indep. Car transfers mod (A) x 1. Community functional transfers require mod (A). Floor transfers dependent. Tub transfers indep c̄ tub bench.

W/C mobility: Indep within facility and in room. Pt requires frequent verbal cues and occasional (A) outside of facility.

Balance: Dynamic sitting balance fair. Pt able to reach objects in w/c about knee height safely. Static sitting balance WFL. Standing balance not tested.

Bed mobility: Rolling (R) and (L) indep. Sit↔supine indep.

Self-care: Pt indep for bathing, dressing, and grooming.

Equipment: Pt has transfer tub bench, hand-held shower, standard w/c, and Jay cushion.

C) What are Kevin's goals?

Kevin would like to return to college in the fall. It is currently May, and he has been accepted into the accounting program at a nearby university. He is concerned that his parents are never going to let him live on his own. Kevin has a girlfriend of 3 years and he is worried that their relationship is not going well. She is currently attending the university where Kevin was accepted. Kevin would like to live in a dorm room with his peers.

Exercise 2:1c

D) How can Kevin reach his goals?

1. Identify Kevin's strengths and weaknesses.

2. Identify the major skills Kevin will need to be able to go back to college. (List long-range goals.)

3. What specific skills and equipment needs will you have to address in order to work toward the major skills listed above? Why? (List short-term goals.)

4. Identify two specific activities per area addressed above in Section 3.

Answers on page 174.

■ Exercise 2:1d—Ethel

A) Where is Ethel now?

Ethel is 79 y/o c̄ a dx of (L) THR. Her medical hx includes: a broken (R) wrist in 1984, a hysterectomy in 1984 that resulted in bladder leakage, high blood pressure, arthritis of (L) knee, and scleroderma on (B) UE. Her precautions include WBAT, no hip √ past 90°, no adduction past neutral. She needs to maintain these precautions for 8 weeks. She is medically stable and will be discharged in 2 weeks.

B) What is Ethel's current status?

Cog status: Intact for orientation and direction following.

UE strength: (L) proximal strength G –; distal G; (R) proximal G –; elbow √ pronation/supination G; wrist/fingers G –.

Transfers: Mod x 2 s̄ ambulation device. Ethel only tolerates minimum weight on her (L) LE during transfer. She requires mod (A) x 1 c̄ walker for 10- to 15- foot distances.

Balance: Static/dynamic sitting balance good, pt able to take full challenges in upright position; reaching past knees not tested 2° to THR precautions.

Bed mobility: Rolling → (R) indep., rolling → (L) indep c̄ c/o pain, sit ↔ supine mod x 1.

UE status: Pt shows bright, shiny skin on (R) palm and about 1/3 of distal forearms. Pt shows multiple bumps in forearm area. Sensation intact. Shoulders and elbows show WFL for AROM (B). (B) hand coordination shows mod ↓'d functioning 2° to poor ability to completely grasp items.

Self-care skills: UE dressing slow but independent. Pt depend for LE dressing 2° to pain and THR precautions. Pt currently dependent for household mobility and requires mod (A) for self-bathing 2° to THR precautions.

Equipment: Pt currently does not have equipment at home.

C) What are Ethel's goals?

Ethel lived at home with her husband prior to this injury. She was independent with her self-care and household responsibilities. Ethel's husband works 3 days a week with their son at a neighborhood store. The business relies on him being there, so he will not be at home with Ethel every day. Ethel wants to return home and be as little burden as possible to her husband.

Exercise 2:1d

D) How can Ethel reach her goals?

1. Identify Ethel's strengths and weaknesses.

2. Identify the major skills Ethel will need in order to reach her goals. (List long-range goals.)

3. What specific skills will you need to address in order to work toward the major skills listed above? Why? (List short-term goals.)

4. Identify two specific activities per area addressed above in Section 3.

Answers on page 175.

■ Exercise 2:1e—Schoci

A) Where is Schoci now?

Schoci is a 53 y/o F with a hx of (L) CVA s/p 2 weeks. She is a very small, thin woman originally from Korea. She does not speak any English. Her nephew is available 2 times per week as an interpreter for the next 2 weeks. She has just been transferred from the acute care floor to a rehabilitation unit for 6 to 8 weeks. There is no other significant medical hx. Schoci lives with her sister and her family. She took care of the three children, cleaned the house, and prepared the meals.

B) What is Schoci's current status?

Orientation: The pt is oriented to person and is able to recognize her relatives, nurses, and therapists. Pt not oriented to time or place.

(R) UE status: UE shows flaccid tone throughout. Shoulder is subluxated 1/2 finger. Pt shows minimum edema in hand and shows facial expression of pain at end ranges of PROM. PROM of UE WFL. No AROM noted with facilitation at this time.

(L) UE status: AROM—WFL, strength fair+, coordination intact. No significant edema or subluxation noted. Normal tone. Pt grip strength 15#.

Posture/head control: WFL actively; pt sits with head turned to the left.

Transfers: Mod x 1 and SBA of another from w/c ↔ mat table.

Balance: Static sitting balance fair. Pt able to sit EOM safely $\bar{s}$ any challenges, such as reaching or pushing on trunk. Dynamic sitting balance poor. Unable to take any challenges to balance. Standing balance poor; pt shows minimum weight bearing on (L) LE during standing.

Bed mobility: Sit ↔ supine mod (A); roll → (R) min (A); roll → (L) max (A).

Sensation: Unable to assess accurately 2° to communication status. Pt responded to light touch stimuli both (R) and (L) UEs and (R) stereognosis appears absent. (L) stereognosis appears intact.

Perception: Pt shows min (R) neglect. Unable to test perception; however, it appears functional during clinical observations.

Communication: Limited to reliable yes/no responses and gestures 2° to language barrier.

Self-care: Pt depend for bathing and dressing. She is able to perform min self-grooming tasks $\bar{c}$ the support of the w/c.

Equipment: Pt currently has no adaptive equipment.

Exercise 2:1e

C) What are Schoci's goals?

According to Korean tradition, when a family member becomes disabled the family is responsible for taking care of him or her. The disabled family member is not expected to contribute to the care and maintenance of himself or herself or the household. Schoci and her family feel very strongly about maintaining this tradition in their household. Schoci will return home to her sister's family and be taken care of, regardless of the level of care she requires.

D) How can Schoci reach her goals?

1. Identify Schoci's strengths and weaknesses.

2. Identify the major skills Schoci or her family will in order for Schoci to go home. (List long-term goals.)

3. What specific skills and equipment needs must be addressed for Schoci to work toward the major skills listed above? Why? (List short-term goals.)

4. Identify two specific activities per area addressed above in Section 3.

Answers on page 176.

To complete the next questions, disregard the family's views on tradition by using the information in Question C below in the place of the preceding information in Question C. Determine how this will change the treatment plan.

C) What are Schoci's goals?

Schoci and her family would like her to return home with her sister's family. She would like to contribute to the household care in some capacity and would like to be as independent as possible.

D) How can Schoci reach these goals?

1. Identify Schoci's strengths and weaknesses.

2. Identify the major skills Schoci and her family will need to enable Schoci to go home. (List long-term goals.)

3. What specific skills and equipment will be needed in order to work toward the major skills listed above? Why? (List short-term goals.)

4. Identify two specific activities per area addressed above in Section 3.

Answers on pages 177–178.

■ Exercise 2:1f—Extra Credit

The therapy plan formula provided can also be useful in setting up goals for an occupational therapy program. By gathering the appropriate information as outlined, this formula can be a very useful tool for determining realistic directions for problem solving in a variety of situations.

Complete Question D in the following exercise using answers like those provided.

A) What is the current situation?

You have just been hired as a consultant in a nursing home two afternoons a week. You are the only OT on staff and there is no formal program in place. There are four nurses' aides assigned to work with you. There are 37 patients in the facility. A regulation body for the nursing home indicates that it must have an active OT program in place to maintain tits license. The nursing home will be reviewed in 3 months.

B) What is the current status?

- Nurses and nurses' aides only provide total care for the residents and have limited knowledge of the function of an OT.
- There are no recreation activities available for the patients.
- There is no OT documentation system in place. (Remember, orders need to be written by a physician to provide OT.)
- There is no formal splint monitoring in place.

C) What does the facility want?

- Formalized recreation activities
- Documentation that patients are being referred appropriately and receiving OT.

D) How would you fulfill the facility goals?

Answers on page 179.

■ Exercise 2:2

Read all the patient information that is provided in each exercise. Complete the questions that follow. You are encouraged to use any occupational therapy references that are available.

■ Exercise 2:2a—Debbie

Debbie is a 39 y/o F in a rehabilitation setting.

Referral reads:

- Dx: (L) CVA
- Provide ADL training and ↑ UE functioning.

Medical chart indicates:

- (L) CVA
- Hypertension

Debbie is in a deltoid aid. This device is used to support the weight of her arm for evaluation and muscle reeducation. Her muscle tone is flaccid to normal.

Figure 2:2a—Debbie

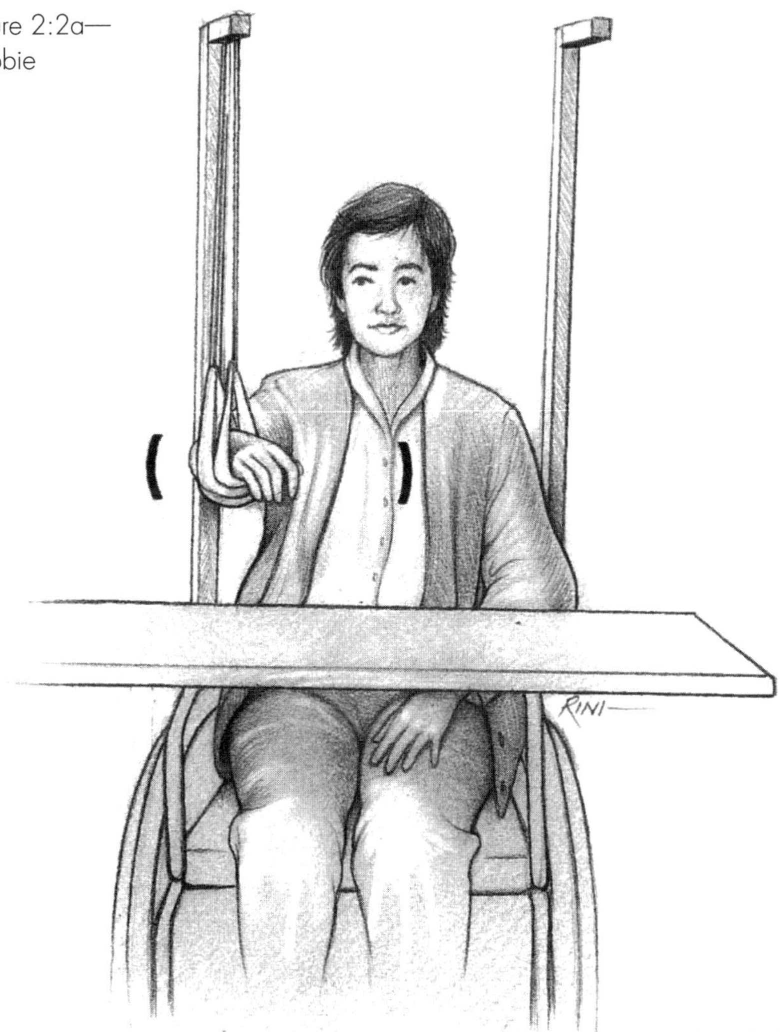

Exercise 2:2a

A) Based on the information given in Figure 2.2a, what are Debbie's AROM planes/patterns at this shoulder? (Assuming there is no movement in her elbow, wrist, or fingers, document her UE AROM as you would a note. Make sure you consider the plane and description of the movement.)

B) Would you identify a strength grade for the muscle movement? If so, what strength grade would you assign?

C) How would you position the patient to determine the other ranges of movement in her left upper extremity?

D) List three ways to facilitate the movement in the shoulder (Debbie can be put in any position).

E) Would you concentrate on working with movement in the hand and fingers now? Why or why not?

F) Formulate two goals related to increasing Debbie's shoulder movement.

Answers on page 180.

■ Exercise 2:2b—Phillip

Phillip is a 9 y/o M admitted to a rehabilitation unit. The average length of stay is 6 months. No significant medical hx prior to injury. Trach tube extubation s/p 2 weeks. Colostomy bag and catheter placed s/p 3 weeks. Frontal and occipital lobe contusion c̄ diffuse lesions.

Referral reads:

- CHI
- Begin eval for ADL.

Medical chart information:

The facility you work in is interdisciplinary. It is common practice to work with the physical therapist on gross motor skills and the speech pathologist on communication skills. Each session is described, including the goals of the physical therapist and the speech pathologist.

Physical therapy and occupational therapy information:

Phillip has been brought to the department on a stretcher. He was a total lift to transfer and he is lying on the mat. His facial expression and increased body tone indicates that he is crying. He appears to be in pain "all over" when you try to move him. Phillip shows flaccid tone throughout his body, except minimum reflexive movement in his upper and lower extremities. He shows minimum head control while sitting edge-of-mat, by moving his head left and right, but he requires a head rest for head support at all times. You and the physical therapist have agreed it is too early to attempt any lower extremity weight-bearing activities at this time.

Physical therapy goals:

- Pt will tolerate PROM to all extremities
- Pt will tolerate sitting EOM with total support for 1 minute

Speech pathology and occupational therapy information:

Phillip is in a reclining w/c. He is unable to speak or move his lips effectively to mouth words. He can use his eyes to look right and left, and identify some pictures and words by eye gaze. He is able to control his eye blinks. Phillip attempts to blow out a match, but his lips are not in the correct position and he has minimum breath support. He cries s̄ sound when he cannot do any task he is asked to do.

Speech therapy goals:

- Patient able to perform oral motor exercises with modeling and visual cues (use of mirror).
- Patient able to identify four needs by using a communication board and eye gazes with set-up.

Occupational therapy goals:

A) Devise goals that take into consideration w/c positioning, tolerance, joint protection of UEs, gross motor movement, and head control.

B)What w/c equipment would you provide for Phillip and what type of tolerance schedule would you attempt?

C) Devise additional goals that take into consideration y/n responses, orientation, possible use of future devices with physical recovery, breath control, and general methods to ease Phillip's fear of the situation.

D) Based on all the goals provided above, identify two activities per goal that will help accomplish the therapy goals during your joint sessions.

1a)

b)

2a)

b)

3a)

b)

4a)

b)

E) How do you explain the situation to Phillip in order to enhance his cooperation with the plan you have outlined?

Answers on page 181.

■ Exercise 2:2—Cooking Group

You would like to organize a cooking group for therapy. There are three patients who the staff agree would be appropriate for the group. Not all the patients are yours, so you have checked with the other therapists and received the information below.

Cheryl:

49 y/o F, mother of 4, pt expressive aphasic, dx (R) CVA

Focus of therapy:

- ↑ standing tolerance
- One-handed activities
- ↑ pt verbal direction following
- ↑ pt (L) UE strength

Warren:

68 y/o M, retired school teacher, dx (R) BKA, has prosthesis, insulin dependent DM

Focus of therapy:

- ↑ household mobility c̄ cane
- ↑ weight shifting on (R) LE
- ↑ standing tolerance

Eleanor:

79 y/o F, homemaker, loves to work in the kitchen, dx Parkinson's disease c̄ dementia

Focus of therapy:

- Following simple repetitive routines
- ↑ use of (B) UEs
- ↑ social involvement and orientation to surroundings

A) Before deciding on the menu, what do you need to consider for the safety of the patients?

B) Which discipline could you consult to assist with the menu and the food portions for each patient?

Figure 2:2c—Cooking Group Kitchen

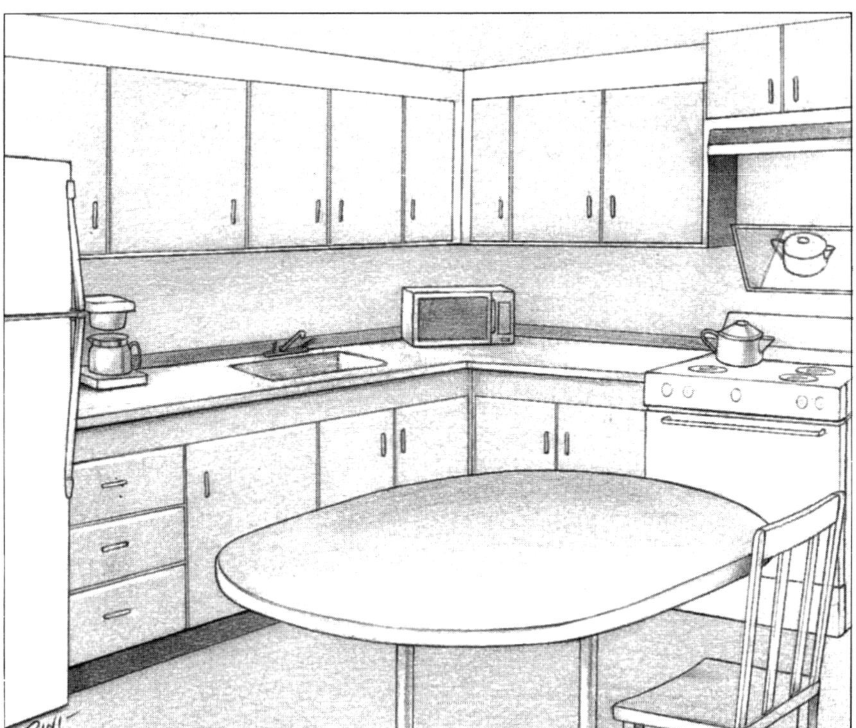

Exercise 2:2c

After consulting with the appropriate discipline, you and the patients have decided on the menu below:

Roasted chicken breast (You have a simple menu card to follow.)

Fresh steamed carrots

Mashed potatoes (You plan on boiling them before the actual meal time.)

Fresh fruit salad (Made with apples, oranges, strawberries, and grapes.)

C) Assign tasks that would be appropriate for each of the patients according to the goals listed above. Not all of the goals have to be addressed, and time is not a factor. Be sure to include tasks such as setting and clearing the table, cleaning up after the meal, and holding appropriately guided table conversations.

D) Formulate one goal for each patient related to the individual's listed deficits and the cooking activity.

Answers on page 182.

■ Exercise 2:2d—Stella

Stella is a 48 y/o F. It is currently June.

Referral reads:

- OT for ADL

Medical chart information:

- (L) CVA
- DM
- Pt married with three children; one daughter lives at home and is currently in high school. Her husband works during the day for a construction company.

Occupational therapy evaluation results:

Interview indicates that pt was independent with ADL prior to incident. She is home alone during the day and does all the cooking and housework. Prior to incident, she used no adaptive equipment.

Sitting balance: G+; pt is able to reach her feet and cross her legs s̄ losing her balance on a firm surface, but has difficulty with these tasks on a soft surface, such as her bed.

Standing balance: F+; pt is able to stand and take minimum challenges, such as perform counter- and table-top activities. Tends to lose her balance when reaching above or below her waist.

(R) UE status: P+ at shoulder, P at elbow/wrist, trace finger movement. PROM is WFL. Pt shows no pain or edema in (R) UE c̄ PROM.

(L) UE strength: AROM is WFL, strength is normal throughout.

Cognitive status: Pt displays no significant language problems. Her memory and judgment are intact. She is able to follow directions appropriately. She is completely oriented, but shows minimum deficits with sequencing ADL tasks.

ADL status: Pt requires moderate (A) donning/doffing her shirt 2° to (↓'d) use of (R) UE and poor sequencing of task. She requires mod (A) to don/doff pants 2° to (↓'d) standing balance and requires moderate (A) to don socks 2° to (↓'d) use of (R) UE. Pt requires minimum (A) to transfer in and out of tub, using transfer tub bench. She requires minimum (A) for bathing. She requires minimum (A) to use WBQC during household mobility 2° to difficulty c̄ dynamic standing balance. Pt requires (A) to reach areas above or below waist during kitchen activities 2° to balance difficulties.

Exercise 2:2d

With the information provided, complete the following two sections.

Part 1:

Stella is in an acute care hospital and will be staying 5 to 7 days. She will be discharged to go home with her husband and daughter.

A) Set up an appropriate therapy plan for Stella's length of stay.

B) What recommendations would you make for discharge?

C) Write three goals for your therapy plan.

Part 2:

Stella is on a rehabilitation unit and will be staying for 5 to 6 weeks.

A) Set up an appropriate therapy plan for Stella's length of stay.

B) Write three goals for your therapy plan.

Answers on page 183.

■ Exercise 2:2e—Peter

Peter is a 73 y/o M c̄ a dx of CVA. April is his occupational therapist. She has been working with Peter for 2 weeks. She is at her desk talking to Sally, another occupational therapist. April tells Sally she does not know what is wrong with Peter.

"He has a lot of potential for recovery, but he will not work on his arm or do any of the perception activities I give him. I try to make the activities interesting. His arm and perception are the only things I am focusing on right now. I guess he is just not motivated to get better," she says.

April has the next day off, and Sally fills in for her and sees Peter. Below are descriptions of the therapy sessions with Peter and each of the therapists.

April and Peter:

April: "Good morning, Peter. Let's work on your arm first today. I thought we would practice bowling since you used to be in a league." (She brings out a small plastic ball and sets up the plastic pins. April has to physically help Peter with all the movement for the activity.)

Peter: "I'm tired. Can we stop?"

April: "Okay, we will rest for a couple of minutes. Then I have a peg design for you to work on."

Peter: "Great!"

Sally and Peter:

Sally: "Good morning, Peter. My name is Sally. April is not here today, so I will be working with you. I see from your treatment plan that you are working on your right arm and perception skills. What would you like to do this morning?"

Peter: "I want to work on my walking. What is 'perception' anyway?"

Sally: "Perception is the ability to understand exactly what you see. For example, if we are both going to walk up a flight of stairs, I might think that the steps are 4 inches high and you might think they are 6 inches high. We both see the steps, but one of us is going to have problems when we try to lift our feet to go up. Now you want to work on walking. Okay. Let's start with standing at the table. You should be able to stand before you can walk." (Sara helps Peter stand at the table using both arms to push up from the w/c.)

Sally: "You stand pretty well. Now let's challenge your balance a little. Pick up these pegs and put them in this basket, first with your left hand, then with your right hand. You should feel your weight shifting from hip, to hip just like walking."

(Peter stands about 10 minutes and uses his left and right hand for the activity. He requires minimum assistance for use of his right hand.)

Sally: "Are you getting tired?" (She feels Peter's hips and knees weakening.)

Peter: "No, I'm fine."

Sally: "Well, I'm getting tired, so let's sit down." (She helps him sit back in the wheelchair using both of his hands to lower himself.) "Now, Peter, remember what I told you about perception and the steps?"

Peter: "Yes, I understand now."

Sally: "Okay. I would like you to copy this block design to work on your ability to trust what you see."

Peter: "Sure."

(Peter finishes the design. Sally assists him with a few corrections.)

Peter: "I guess I do have a problem with that. Thanks, Sally, and I'll see you this afternoon."

A) Did both April and Sally work on the same goals for Peter?

B) Were the activities developed by April inappropriate for his skill level?

C) Why did Sally get such a different response from Peter?

D) Does Peter have a motivation problem? If not, why was April having such a difficult time with Peter?

E) If you were Sally, would you say anything to April? If so, what would you say?

F) Does a patient have the right not to work on a specific area of dysfunction, even if he or she has good potential for recovery?

Answers on page 184.

■ Exercise 2:2f—Mark

Mark is sitting on the edge of the mat working with a set of pegs at a table. The pegs are 1 inch in diameter and they are different colors. They fit in a board with precarved holes. He is taking the pegs out of a bucket and placing them on the board. Based on the information provided in each section below, describe how you would alter this task to challenge each deficit listed by answering the following questions. Other pieces of therapeutic equipment can be added to the tasks.

Figure 2.2f—Mark

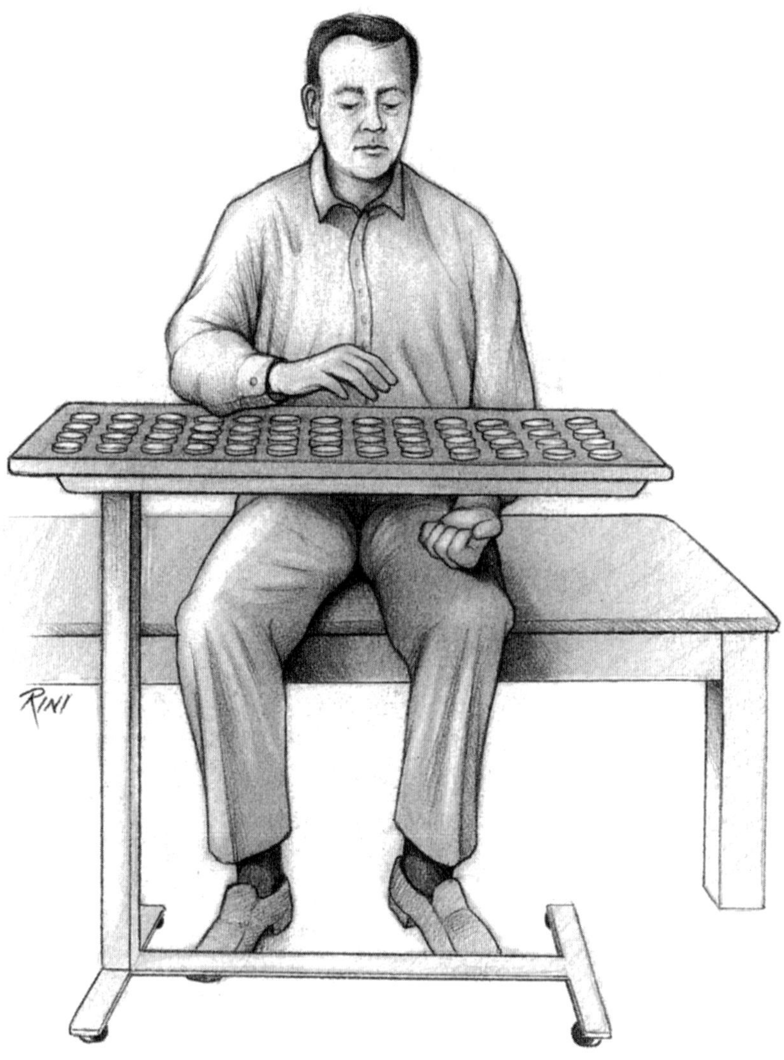

Part 1:

Mark is working on sitting balance. He is able to sit comfortably on the edge of the mat and do this activity.

A) How would you upgrade the activity?

B) Formulate one goal related to the task.

Part 2:

Mark is working on strengthening his left upper extremity. His arm can comfortably perform this activity.

A) How would you upgrade this activity?

B) Formulate one goal related to the task.

Part 3:

Mark is very confused and unable to sequence simple tasks. He is able to follow directions for the activity listed above by just picking and placing random pegs.

A) How would you upgrade this activity?

B) Formulate one goal related to the task.

Answers on page 185.

■ Exercise 2:2g—Mabel

Mabel is 68 years old. She has a diagnosis of a hip fracture and she has a medical history of dementia. Mabel has been living with her daughter and son-in-law for the past 3 years. During her initial OT evaluation, you ask Mabel to raise her arms. She is not able to raise them. Then you give her a towel and ask her to fold it. She folds it perfectly, including shaking it out. You ask her to stand up. She tries, but is unable to coordinate the movements to stand. You ask her to get some butter out of the refrigerator. She stands up but requires minimum assistance to walk to the refrigerator. Mabel is not able to follow directions, but she can perform spontaneous functional activities. She has no medical restrictions, and yet shows discomfort when bending to touch her feet.

A) When you form your therapy plan, do you include a goal that states Mabel will be able to follow commands? Why or why not? (Review functional deficits as a result of dementia.)

B) Assuming you have an apartment set-up and any equipment you need, list three activities for each goal listed below.

Pt able to perform functional transfers for everyday living independently.

1.

2.

3.

Pt able to stand with minimum challenges and equal weight bearing on LEs for 10 minutes. (Assume minimum challenge is moving arms between shoulder and waist height.)

1.

2.

3.

Pt able to don/doff shoes and socks $\bar{c}$ SBA. (Analyze the movements needed for this activity in relation to the injury.)

1.

2.

3.

Answers on page 186.

■ Exercise 2:2h—Bob

Bob is a 58-year-old male who suffered a CVA 5 days ago. He is a large man. His hobbies include fishing, hunting, and working on cars. He was employed as a foreman at a car factory. Bob was very active; his wife says he was never home because he always found something to do. Bob is expressively and receptively aphasic. He has Fair– strength on the right side of his body. He has come to the department for the first time in a wheelchair. You introduce yourself. Bob cries very hard and points to his mouth and hand.

A) What do you say or do? How would you explain to him what happened and why he is here to see you? (Remember, he is aphasic, so any explanations need to be short phrases and gestures.)

B) Based on the information provided above, for Bob's therapy plan, would you focus on increasing his independence or redeveloping his functional abilities? For example, would you teach him one-handed dressing or work on developing functional reeducation of his arm, or both? Why?

Answers on page 187.

■ Exercise 2:2i—Eleanor

Eleanor is a 79-year-old woman who suffered a left CVA 7 days ago. She is brought to the department in a wheelchair. Her head is positioned severely to the right. You begin your initial interview with her, and she suddenly stops and leans very close to you. She says, "I think I am losing my mind." A tear slides down her cheek. She continues, "I am hearing voices." With further questioning, you find out that when people talk to her on her left side or the left side of the room, she does not turn her head. Her hospital bed is by the window, and she is not aware that she has a roommate in the bed to her left.

A) Before you continue with the evaluation process, Eleanor will need to be able to deal with her current concerns. What could be the reason for her concerns?

B) How do you explain this situation to her? (Remember to explain it to her in terms she can understand.)

C) Is there anything you can suggest that will make her more comfortable in her room?

Answers on page 188.

■ Exercise 2:2j—Dr. Bones

Dr. Bones, a psychiatrist, has been referred to the OT department after a THR. He has been retired for about 3 years.

Dr. Bones: "What exactly did they do to me?"

A) You reply:

Dr. Bones: "What am I doing here?"

B) You reply:

Answers on page 189.

■ Exercise 2:2k—Toni

Toni is a 17-year-old girl who was involved in a motor vehicle accident. A summary of her OT evaluation is complete, and the results are listed below. There is a family meeting scheduled for Toni, and you need to report the results of your evaluation and your therapy plan.

Evaluation Results:

Pt unable to sit EOM 2° to poor trunk control. She requires support of one person to maintain sitting balance on unsupported surfaces. Pt requires max x 2 to transfer w/c ↔ mat. She shows poor movement in (L) shoulder and no movement at elbow/wrist/fingers. Pt has difficulty following directions 2° to receptive deficits. She is able to understand gestures, imitate movements, and understand simple one-step commands.

Therapy Plan:

- Plan to ↑ trunk stability to tolerate sitting EOM $\bar{s}$ support.
- Plan to ↑ transfers to mod x 1 for w/c ↔ mat transfers.
- Facilitate movement of (L) UE to be used as a functional assist during activities.
- ↑ pt's ability to follow directions during functional tasks.

Determine what you would say to the family in the following situations. In all cases remember to watch the terminology you use and try to relate the explanations to situations the patient's family can understand as much as possible. The order in which you present information can help in more delicate situations.

Situation A:

Toni's mother has never worked outside the home. She has a junior high level education. Her father is a linesman in a factory. Both appear ready to accept any deficits their daughter has and are ready to help her get better.

Situation B:

Toni's mother is a nurse who has been working on an orthopedic floor for 5 years. Her father is a businessman and travels a great deal. Both are very worried about how they can manage a disabled daughter at home.

Situation C:

Toni's mother is an accountant and her father is a lawyer. The mother is very quiet and appears to not be paying attention to anything. The father is very close to his daughter and cries frequently.

Situation A:

Situation B:

Situation C:

Answers on page 190.

■ Exercise 2:2L—Alan

Alan is 48 years old. He has had a BKA of the left lower extremity and has received his prosthesis. He is a stockbroker, and during the initial interview appeared very anxious to get back to work. He has told you about a pain he has been feeling in his left foot and leg. He says, "I know that is ridiculous since my leg is gone, but it really hurts."

A) How would you explain phantom pain to Alan?

B) Alan also asks, "Why do I need to waste my time here anyway?" What do you say to him?

C) If Alan were 6 years old and crying, how would you explain phantom pain to him?

Answers on page 191.

■ Exercise 2:2m—Gerry

Gerry is 27 years old. He is mentally retarded and has lived with his parents all of his life. He is functioning at a 5-year-old developmental level. Gerry had an MI 4 days ago and has been referred to OT for evaluation.

A) Gerry looks scared and asks, "Where is my mommy?" What would you tell him?

B) Gerry asks, "What happened to me? Why am I here?" How would you explain the situation to him?

Answers on page 192.

■ Exercise 2:2n—Joe

Joe is 27 years old. His diagnosis is multiple gunshot wounds with an incomplete T-5–T-6 and head injury. Joe is 6'2", 230 pounds, and has a 6th-grade education. As you approach the nursing station and pull the chart, the nurse says, "That man is wild; he yells and curses at everyone. He has been cussing the doctors and nurses out for the last 3 days. Good luck."

The social history indicates he has been working on a loading dock for 8 months and has a girlfriend. There are also indications of drug and alcohol abuse.

A) Knowing Joe's history and his current situation, what are possible causes for his behavior?

B) As you enter the room, Joe is lying in bed staring out the window. How do you introduce yourself and explain OT?

C) What areas do you think would be appropriate to begin with for your evaluation?

Answers on page 193.

■ Exercise 2:2o—Jessica

Jessica is a 10-year-old girl with a diagnosis of CHI due to a motor vehicle accident. She has been in a rehabilitation unit for 4 months. She is currently able to use her right hand to operate a joystick on computer games without difficulty; however, she is not able to use grasp or release, or to hold a pencil. She remains very flaccid throughout her body and may have the potential to walk, but only with years of continued therapy. Her cognitive functioning is within functional limits for her age.

About a month ago, you, as her occupational therapist, felt that she could successfully benefit from an electric wheelchair. Jessica also saw a patient with an electric wheelchair and has been asking you what she has to be able to do in order to have a chair like that. You discussed the subject with her father and mother. Her father was very angry with the idea, and her mother was very quiet.

The next day Jessica and her father came down to therapy, and Jessica said, "I don't want an electric wheelchair. I will be walking soon." The entire rehabilitation team feels that Jessica can begin school in August with the correct equipment.

A) Why did Jessica's father become angry?

B) Would you address the issue of the electric wheelchair with this family again?

C) If you did, what would you say and how would you say it?

D) Would you get Jessica involved in the process of deciding about the wheelchair? If so, when?

E) Based on the assumption that the right arm movement is the only controllable movement Jessica has, what other equipment ideas could you suggest for going back to school?

Answers on page 194.

■ Exercise 2:2p—Terri

Terri is a 32-year-old woman with a diagnosis of an aneurysm that burst 4 days ago. She is a mother of 2 daughters; one is 5 years old and the other is 2 years old. She is a homemaker and does volunteer work for the local hospital. She prides herself on being able to entertain for her husband's business associates. Terri comes to the department in a reclining chair. She is trying to sit up, yet has no control of her trunk or the right side of her body. She is scared and crying frantically. She appears to understand everything she is told.

A) How do you react to Terri when you first meet her?

B) Explain what is happening to her.

C) Explain why she can't sit up or use her right arm.

D) Explain what you will be doing in therapy and why. (Be careful not to build up false hope or unrealistic expectations.)

Answers on page 195.

■ Exercises 3:1

Read each patient description carefully. Answer the questions that follow each one. You are encouraged to use any occupational therapy references that are available.

■ Exercise 3:1a—Clifford

Clifford is 68 y/o. He suffered a (R) CVA. He is a retired airplane pilot. Clifford is married and has two grown daughters who live in the same township. He enjoys golfing and spending time with his family. Clifford also enjoys visiting in his neighborhood.

Phase of rehabilitation:

Clifford is in a hospital rehabilitation unit. He has been receiving 3 hours of intensive rehab services a day for the past 8 weeks.

Living situation:

Clifford lives c̄ his wife in a one-floor, two-bedroom home. His wife has no significant physical or cognitive limitations. Prior to his CVA, Clifford spent a great deal of time visiting his friends in the neighborhood.

Current status:

Clifford is ambulating short distances c̄ a small-base quad cane. His (L) UE has shown progressive recovery, from being flaccid to Clifford being able to use it as a gross (A). He requires min SBA for bathing and dressing c̄ the use of a transfer tub bench. Clifford has no significant cognitive deficits. His memory, judgment, and safety skills are intact.

Reimbursement options:

Home health care

Continued rehabilitation inpatient care

Outpatient

Long-term care

Exercise 3:1a

A) In your opinion, would Clifford benefit from further occupational therapy rehabilitation services?

B) What level of care would you recommend?

C) Provide an outline for a therapy plan you would recommend for the next level of rehabilitative services that you choose.

D) Would you recommend any type of community programs for Clifford and his family?

Answers on page 197.

■ Exercise 3:1b—Bill

Bill is 53 y/o. He had an aneurysm that burst 2 weeks ago. Bill is married c̄ 2 sons and a daughter. He enjoys fishing and bowling. Bill works in construction. Both he and his wife are very active in their church community.

Phase of rehabilitation:

Bill is in an acute care hospital. He has just become medically stable and is being transferred out of the intensive care unit. He has received OT and PT services.

Living situation:

Bill lives c̄ his wife in a second-floor apartment. His wife is a very petite woman c̄ mild arthritis in her hands. Bill managed all the household finances.

Current status:

Bill has been medically stable for 2 days. He is alert for about a 1/2 hr at a time, but is disoriented and confused. He is beginning to tolerate sitting up on the side of the bed and showing some isolated finger movement in his affected UE. Bill can tolerate doing exercises supine for about 15 minutes c̄ his unaffected UE and LE. The OT and PT working with Bill have decided to begin getting him up in a w/c.

Reimbursement options:

Home health

Inpatient rehabilitation

Long-term care

Exercise 3:1b

A) In your opinion, would Bill benefit from further occupational therapy rehabilitative services?

B) What level of care would you recommend?

C) Provide an outline for a therapy plan that you would recommend for the next level of rehabilitative services you choose.

D) Would you recommend any type of community programs to the patient and his family?

Answers on page 198.

■ Exercise 3:1c—Valerie

Valerie is 36 y/o. She was hit by a car 8 weeks ago. She suffered fractures of the (R) femur and (R) radius, and has a crushed (R) wrist. She is a wife and mother of 2 children; Sarah who is 8 y/o and Nick who is 10 y/o. Valerie enjoys being a homemaker. She also enjoys sewing and needlework.

Phase of recovery:

Valerie has been in a rehabilitation center for 2 weeks. She has been receiving OT and PT services 2 x a day.

Living situation:

Valerie lives c̄ her family. Her sister lives a block away and has been caring for Valerie's children while she has been in the hospital. Valerie's sister is prepared to help her with the transition to home. Valerie's home has two levels and a basement. The bedrooms and bathroom are on the second floor, and the laundry facilities are in the basement.

Current status:

Valerie's femur is healing well. She is ambulating without an assistive device, but she still has difficulty manipulating the stairs ,due to a walking cast. Valerie has had two surgeries on her wrist since the accident. Her wrist cast has been removed, and the physician has ordered AROM as the pt tolerates. Valerie is indep c̄ bathing, dressing, and most other ADL skills, using adaptive techniques learned in OT.

Reimbursement Options:

Home health

Outpatient services

Reentry programs

Exercise 3:1c

A) In your opinion, would Valerie benefit from further occupational therapy rehabilitative services?

B) What level of care would you recommend?

C) Provide an outline for a therapy plan that you would recommend for the next level of rehabilitative services that you choose.

D) Would you recommend any type of community programs to the patient and her family?

Answers on page 199.

Exercise 3:1d—Imogene

Imogene is 83 y/o. Two weeks ago, she fell in her home and broke her hip. She underwent a THR surgical procedure. Imogene has four children who have their own families and live out of town. She is a retired homemaker and her husband passed away 8 years ago. When Imogene was asked about her interests, she said she kept busy. However, she was not able to identify any of her specific interests or hobbies.

Phase of recovery:

Imogene is receiving rehab services in a skilled nursing facility. She is being seen by a PT and an OT.

Living situation:

Imogene lives alone in her two-story home. Her children keep in touch c̄ her by telephone, and two of her daughters visit about 1 week a year. One daughter explained that every visit her mom gets older, but she is still managing to take care of herself. The social worker contacted one of Imogene's neighbors. The neighbor indicated that Imogene has been keeping to herself the last couple of years, and that she has been checking on Imogene regularly. The social worker indicated that Imogene's children would not be able to assist in providing care for her.

Current status:

Imogene is using a walker to ambulate. She is physically able to prepare simple meals. The OT has been teaching her to bathe and dress herself c̄ adaptive equipment so she can maintain her hip precautions for the next 3 weeks. Imogene had a great deal of difficulty learning the new tasks, and her safety awareness and judgment are very poor. The nursing staff reports that in the evening, Imogene becomes very confused and it is difficult to calm her. The physician has indicated that Imogene has the initial symptoms of dementia.

Reimbursement options:

Home health

Long-term care

Outpatient services

Exercise 3:1d

A) In your opinion, would Imogene benefit from further occupational therapy rehabilitative services?

B) What level of care would you recommend?

C) Provide an outline for a therapy plan that you would recommend for the next level of rehabilitative services you choose.

D) Would you recommend any type of community programs to the patient and her family?

Answers on page 200.

■ Exercise 3:1e—Alice

Alice is 20 y/o. She was involved in a diving accident that left her a paraplegic. Prior to her injury, she was very independent. She lived on her own and was working her way through college to be a pharmacist. She was employed as a waitress. Alice enjoys going to school and swimming.

Living situation:

Alice lived alone in an apartment prior to her injury. The injury occurred 4 months ago. Since then, her parents and sister moved her belongings to her parents' home. Alice's parents live in the family home, and her sister has an apartment c̄ a roommate.

Phase of recovery:

Alice is in an inpatient rehab center that specializes in spinal cord–injury recovery. Alice has received services c̄ OT, PT, and a psychologist.

Current status:

Alice is independent c̄ her self-care, transfers, and mobility in a lightweight w/c. Her strength and endurance are good. She has been reviewing her textbooks to catch up c̄ her studies, and plans to return to school in 6 months.

Reimbursement options:

Home health services

Reentry programs

Outpatient services

Exercise 3:1e

A) In your opinion, would Alice benefit from further occupational therapy rehabilitative services?

B) What level of care would you recommend?

C) Provide an outline for a therapy plan that you would recommend for the next level of rehabilitative services you choose.

D) Would you recommend any type of community programs to the patient and her family?

Answers on page 201.

■ Exercise 3:1f—Homer

Homer is 61 y/o. He had a heart attack 2 years ago, and he has DM. Four weeks ago, he had a BKA. Homer has always been very active. Prior to his heart attack, he worked as a salesman and did a lot of traveling. Since his heart attack, he decreased his travel schedule and volunteered as a radio operator for the fire department.

Phase of recovery:

Homer has been receiving OT and PT services in an amputee clinic for 3 weeks.

Living situation:

Homer lives $\bar{c}$ his wife in a one-floor condominium. They have a son who has a family and a home. Homer helps his wife $\bar{c}$ some of the household chores and takes care of the yard duties. Homer's wife is concerned about Homer's reaction to the amputation. He has indicated to her that he is useless $\bar{s}$ his leg, even for volunteer work.

Current status:

Homer has received a LE prosthesis. He is ambulating independently $\bar{c}$ a cane. He is indep $\bar{c}$ dressing, bathing, and transfers $\bar{c}$ his prosthesis. Homer is showing good weight shifting ability, and he is able to monitor his stump skin condition. He went home on a weekend pass and reported he had no difficulties $\bar{c}$ ambulating and self-care.

Reimbursement Options:

Home health services

Reentry programs

Long-term care

A) In your opinion, would Homer benefit from further occupational therapy rehabilitative services?

B) What level of care would you recommend?

C) Provide an outline for a therapy plan you would recommend for the next level of rehabilitative services you choose.

D) Would you recommend any type of community programs to the patient and his family?

Answers on page 202.

■ Exercises 3:2

Read the patient information carefully. Devise a home program for each individual. You are encouraged to use any occupational therapy references that are available.

■ Exercise 3:2a—Ruth

Ruth has a diagnosis of RA. She is having difficulty c̄ her hands and made an appointment c̄ her physician. The physician sent her to the OT clinic c̄ the following referral:

Provide (B) hand splints to be worn nightly and education for joint protection.

A) What areas of therapy would need to be included in the home program?

B) Write a home program for Ruth.

Answers on page 203.

■ Exercise 3:2b—Barbara

Barbara was involved in an accident at an assembly factory. She required surgical repair of both flex and extensor tendons on her (L) hand involving the second and third digits. The physician has sent her to the OT clinic $\bar{c}$ the following referral:

Provide splint for protection, AROM exercise program, no PROM, education for scar massage and edema control.

A) What areas of therapy would need to be included in the home program?

B) Write a home program for Barbara.

Answers on pages 204–205.

Exercise 1:1—Record A

1. **(Answer provided)**

2. **Assessment**

Relevance:

- May need to adjust method of eval or tx to compensate poor endurance.
- Will need an endurance program as part of tx plan.

3. **Assessment**

Relevance:

- Will need to adjust methods for eval or tx to accommodate for the pt's inability to make his wants and needs understood.
- Tx plan or eval can include addressing an appropriate communication system or method.

4. **Objective**

Relevance:

- Indicates a compromised respiratory status that suggests low endurance for activity.

5. **Subjective**

Relevance:

- Father's view of daughter is unrealistic and he may not be able to accept the drinking hx. This information is important for developing an appropriate technique in providing family education with father.

6. **Objective**

Relevance:

- Will need to look further for precautions during tx or eval. Will need to monitor for edema and any joint complications related to injury.

7. **Plan**

Relevance:

- Will need to monitor the pt's weight-bearing status during eval and tx.
- Will need to teach compensation for the non-weight bearing precautions during ADL activity.

8. **Assessment**

Relevance:

- Will be able to set up an eval and tx program that can prepare the pt for an in-depth recovery or compensation plan rather than a short-term program.

9. **Objective**

Relevance:

- Identification of the infarct or lesion location can determine what areas of function are most likely to be affected. Evaluation and/or tx can start with these identified functions.

10. **Plan**

Relevance:

- Will not need to work on eval or adaptation of computer because it has been completed.
- May want to provide cotreatment of support tx in the OT sessions.
- Direction for adaptation to avocational skill development has been determined.

11. **Subjective**

Relevance:

- Pt is unreliable for hx information and orientation. Will need to rely on other resources to receive appropriate information.

12. **Subjective**

Relevance:

- A brief feeding evaluation is needed rather than a thorough evaluation.

13. **Plan**

Relevance:

- Indicated urinary tract infection. The pt may have discomfort in lower back and may need to urinate frequently.

14. **Assessment**

Relevance:

- Provides a guideline for what areas of function should be evaluated.

Exercise 1:1—Record B

1. **(Answer provided)**
2. **Assessment**

Relevance:

- Need to make adjustments in evaluation and treatment techniques to accommodate for the pt's inability to understand verbal directions and speech.

3. **Subjective**

Relevance:

- Indicates pt may have deficits of orientation to time or difficulty c̄ expression. This information helps identify areas to evaluate.

4. **Plan**

Relevance:

- Indicates the direction or focus of tx for sessions.

5. **Subjective**

Relevance:

- Indicates the mood level of the pt that the therapist will encounter during tx and/or evaluation.

6. **Objective**

Relevance:

- Provides a guide to where to begin the evaluation process and what areas of treatment should be addressed.

7. **Assessment**

Relevance:

- Indicates that other resources will need to be accessed for reliable life hx of pt.

8. **Plan**

Relevance:

- Provides a guide for the functional level the pt or husband will need to achieve to reach the discharge goal.
- Provides the family's or pt's view of the current situation. If the pt's prognosis is poor for returning home c̄ her husband, family education will need to be provided to adjust their perception of the situation.

9. **Plan**

Relevance:

- Becoming aware of the bowel and bladder training being initiated allows the other therapists an opportunity to assist c̄ the plan by adjusting their tx plans or being aware that the pt may ask or need to be asked about using the bathroom during tx.

10. **Assessment**

Relevance:

- Indicates that the pt should be evaluated for other types of mobility options (e.g., wheelchair).
- Since the therapist is involved c̄ pts and family education, this information can be reinforced.

11. **Objective**

Relevance:

- The treatment plan can be adjusted to incorporate ambulation c̄ the walker (e.g., household mobility).
- Indicates the amount of assistance the pt needs for ambulation.

12. **Subjective**

Relevance:

- The method of evaluation and treatment techniques will need to be modified to build rapport and not cause the pt discomfort.

13. **Objective or assessment**

Relevance:

- Provides the therapist with information that can be used to approach the pt c̄ eval and tx information.

14. **Subjective**

Relevance:

- Information is used as pt's goal.

15. **Objective**

Relevance:

- Provides information about pt's limitations that is used to develop the treatment plan.

Exercise 1:2—Patient B

A) Diagnosis:

- Anatomy of hand leaves little room for scarring $\bar{s}$ disrupting gliding mechanisms, which can cause ↓ ROM.
- Area of the flexor tendon repair determines the appropriate positioning for splinting.
- Exercises should not permit active finger flexion or passive extension.

  Reference: Trombly, C.A. (1989). *Occupational therapy for physical dysfunction* (3rd ed.) Baltimore: Williams & Wilkins.

B) Phase of recovery:

- Acute because of instability of flexor tendon and precautions.

C) Facility considerations:

- Pt seen 3 x a week as outpatient.

D) Other significant areas:

- Cognitive status for understanding and following directions.

See the following Evaluation Checklist for Patient B.

Category	Rating			Comments
	R	SR	N/A	
A. Independent Living/Daily Living Skills				
Physical Daily Living Skills				
Grooming and Hygiene		X		To indicate if patient requires assistance with one-handed tasks
Feeding/Eating		X		Same as above
Dressing		X		Same as above
Functional Mobility				
Bed Mobility			X	Area not affected by current diagnosis
W/C Mobility			X	Same as above
Transfers			X	Same as above
Functional Ambulation			X	Same as above
Functional Communication			X	Same as above
Object Manipulation			X	Same as above
Psychological/Emotional Daily Living Skills				
Self-Concept/Self-Identity			X	
Situational Coping		X		To identify the patient's ability to cope with situations
Community Involvement			X	
Work				
Homemaking		X		To indicate if the patient requires assistance with one-handed tasks
Child Care/Parenting		X		Same as above
Employment Preparation			X	Too soon to address after injury
Play/Leisure			X	

Evaluation Checklist

Patient Name: Patient B

LEGEND: R—RELEVANT; SR—SOMEWHAT RELEVANT; N/A—NOT APPLICABLE

Category	Rating			Comments
	R	SR	N/A	
B. Sensorimotor Components				
Neuromuscular				
Reflex Integration			X	No neurological involvement
Range of Motion				
PROM			X	By physician's order
AROM	X			Establish baseline information
A/AROM			X	By physician's order
Gross and Fine Coordination				
Muscle Control	X			Gross muscle control as baseline for evaluation
Coordination	X			Gross coordination as baseline for evaluation
Dexterity			X	Not appropriate for acute phase
Strength and Endurance			X	Same as above
Sensory Integration			X	Area not affected
Sensory Awareness	X			Gross sensory evaluation in affected areas
Visual-Spatial Awareness			X	Area not affected
Body Integration				
Body Schema			X	Area not affected
Postural Balance			X	Same as above
(B) Motor Coordination			X	Not appropriate for acute phase
Right-Left Discrimination			X	Area not affected
Visual-Motor Integration			X	Same as above
Crossing Midline			X	Same as above
Praxis			X	Same as above
C. Cognitive Components				
Orientation			X	Area not affected
Conceptualization/Comprehension	X			To ensure patient is able to understand and follow home program

Evaluation Checklist continued

Patient Name: Patient B

LEGEND: R—RELEVANT; SR—SOMEWHAT RELEVANT; N/A—NOT APPLICABLE

Category	Rating			Comments
	R	SR	N/A	
Concentration		X		To ensure patient is able to understand and follow home program
Attention Span		X		Same as above
Memory		X		Same as above
Cognitive Integration				
Generalizing			X	
Problem Solving		X		To ensure patient is able to understand and follow home program
Defining or Evaluating a Problem			X	
Organizing a Plan			X	
Implementing a Plan		X		
Evaluating a Decision			X	
D. Psychosocial Components				
Self-Management				
Self-Expression		X		To determine patient's ability to communicate concerns
Self-Control			X	Not an affected area
Dyadic Interaction		X		To determine patient's ability to communicate concerns
Group Interaction			X	No application in situation and not affected area
E. Therapeutic Adaptations				
Orthotics	X			As ordered by physician
Prosthetics			X	
Assistive/Adaptive Equipment		X		May need devices or education in one-handed devices
F. Prevention				
Energy Conservation			X	Not affected area
Joint Protection/Body Mechanics	X			Protect hand during recovery
Positioning	X			Splint and edema positioning
Coordination of Daily Living Activities		X		If needed to manage one-handed activities

Evaluation Checklist continued

Patient Name: Patient B

LEGEND: R—RELEVANT; SR—SOMEWHAT RELEVANT; N/A—NOT APPLICABLE

Evaluation chart adapted from the *Reference Manual of the Official Documents of the American Occupational Therapy Association, Inc.* (pp. VIII.22–23) by The American Occupational Therapy Association, 1986, Rockville, MD: Author.

Exercise 1:2—Patient C

A) Diagnosis:

Parkinson's Disease:

- Characteristics—rigidity, tremor, and bradykinesia.
- ↓ in activity of the neurotransmitter dopamine in the basal ganglia.
- Parkinsonian–dementia complex.

Treatment:

- Levadopa—L-Dopa crosses the blood–brain barrier and enters the central nervous system (CNS) where it undergoes enzymatic conversion to dopamine.

Reference: Gilroy, J., & Holliday, P.L. (1982). *Basic neurology* (p.104).New York: Macmillan.

Commonly used evaluations include:

- ROM
- Muscle tone
- Righting reactions
- Speed and accuracy of voluntary movements
- Automatic postural movements
- ADL status

Ongoing evaluation to provide feedback to the physician to gauge effectiveness of medication levels.

Reference: Trombly, C.A. (1989). *Occupational therapy for physical dysfunction* (3rd ed.). Baltimore: Williams & Wilkins.

B) Phase of recovery:

- Postacute because she is medically stable.

C) Facility considerations:

- Acute care hospital
- 1 wk LOS
- Pt seen 1 hr per day

D) Other significant areas:

- Family's report of confusion
- Her age (78 y/o)
- Functional level prior to incident

See the following Evaluation Checklist for Patient C.

Category	Rating			Comments
	R	SR	N/A	
A. Independent Living/Daily Living Skills				
Physical Daily Living Skills				
Grooming and Hygiene	X			Patient returning home alone; requires physical and cognitive ability
Feeding/Eating	X			Same as above
Dressing	X			Same as above
Functional Mobility				
Bed Mobility	X			Patient returning home alone; requires physical and cognitive ability
W/C Mobility		X		Applicable if patient has wheelchair
Transfers	X			Patient returning home alone; requires physical and cognitive ability
Functional Ambulation	X			Same as above
Functional Communication		X		Area not directly affected by diagnosis, but questionable secondary to confusion
Object Manipulation	X			Relates to patient's motor skills affected by diagnosis
Psychological/Emotional Daily Living Skills				
Self-Concept/Self-Identity		X		
Situational Coping	X			To determine patient's ability to live alone
Community Involvement	X			Same as above
Work				
Homemaking	X			To determine patient's ability to live alone
Child Care/Parenting			X	Patient lives alone
Employment Preparation			X	Patient is retired
Play/Leisure		X		Address if able to in short period of time

Evaluation Checklist

Patient Name: Patient C

LEGEND: R—RELEVANT; SR—SOMEWHAT RELEVANT; N/A—NOT APPLICABLE

Category	Rating			Comments
	R	SR	N/A	
B. Sensorimotor Components				
Neuromuscular				
Reflex Integration	X			Righting reactions for safety and automatic postural movements
Range of Motion				
PROM	X			Determine baseline and progress
AROM	X			Same as above
A/AROM	X			Same as above
Gross and Fine Coordination				
Muscle Control	X			Determine baseline and progress
Coordination	X			Same as above
Dexterity	X			Same as above
Strength and Endurance	X			Same as above
Sensory Integration			X	Area not affected by diagnosis
Sensory Awareness		X		May be problem secondary to diagnosis or age
Visual-Spatial Awareness			X	Area not affected by diagnosis
Body Integration				
Body Schema			X	Area not affected by diagnosis
Postural Balance	X			Relevant for safety and affected by diagnosis
(B) Motor Coordination	X			Same as above
Right-Left Discrimination			X	Area not affected by diagnosis
Visual-Motor Integration			X	Same as above
Crossing Midline			X	Same as above
Praxis			X	Same as above
C. Cognitive Components				
Orientation	X			Areas could be affected by diagnosis or age; patient lives alone
Conceptualization/Comprehension	X			Same as above

Evaluation Checklist continued

Patient Name: Patient C

LEGEND: R—RELEVANT; SR—SOMEWHAT RELEVANT; N/A—NOT APPLICABLE

Category	Rating			Comments
	R	SR	N/A	
Concentration	X			Areas could be affected by diagnosis or age; patient lives alone
Attention Span	X			Same as above
Memory	X			Same as above
Cognitive Integration				
Generalizing	X			Areas could be affected by diagnosis or age; patient lives alone
Problem Solving	X			Same as above
Defining or Evaluating a Problem	X			Same as above
Organizing a Plan	X			Same as above
Implementing a Plan	X			Same as above
Evaluating a Decision	X			Same as above
D. Psychosocial Components				
Self-Management				
Self-Expression		X		
Self-Control			X	Areas not affected by diagnosis
Dyadic Interaction			X	Same as above
Group Interaction			X	Same as above
E. Therapeutic Adaptations				
Orthotics			X	Same as above
Prosthetics			X	Same as above
Assistive/Adaptive Equipment		X		May be relevant if patient has difficulty with freedom of movement
F. Prevention				
Energy Conservation		X		May be relevant depending on physical or cognitive status
Joint Protection/Body Mechanics			X	Area not relevant for diagnosis
Positioning		X		If patient is still rigid, may need assistance with chair types
Coordination of Daily Living Activities		X		May need education or assistance, depending on cognitive and physical status

Evaluation Checklist continued

Patient Name: Patient C

LEGEND: R—RELEVANT; SR—SOMEWHAT RELEVANT; N/A—NOT APPLICABLE

Evaluation chart adapted from the *Reference Manual of the Official Documents of the American Occupational Therapy Association, Inc.* (pp. VIII.22–23) by The American Occupational Therapy Association, 1986, Rockville, MD: Author.

Exercise 1:2—Patient D

A) Diagnosis:

Spina Bifida

- Varying degrees of incomplete bony closure of one or more neural arches. Most frequent site is the lumbosacral region.
- Neurological deficits can vary from mild muscle imbalance and sensory loss in lower limbs to complete paraplegia.
- Possible bowel and bladder disruption.

Reference: Salter, R.B. (1983). *Textbook of disorders and injuries of the musculoskeletal system* (pp. 132–136). Baltimore: Williams & Wilkins.

B) Phase of recovery:

- Postacute or rehabilitation because pt is medically stable and therapeutic intervention is needed for effective mainstreaming into the school system.

C) Facility considerations:

- Student to be seen 1 x per week.

D) Other significant areas:

- The child's age and her developmental progression status may have been influenced by her limitations or past environments.

See the following Evaluation Checklist for Patient D.

Category	Rating			Comments
	R	SR	N/A	
A. Independent Living/Daily Living Skills				
Physical Daily Living Skills				
Grooming and Hygiene	X			Specifically bowel & bladder care secondary to diagnosis
Feeding/Eating			X	
Dressing	X			Specifically lower extremity dressing secondary to diagnosis
Functional Mobility				
Bed Mobility		X		To provide training for parent follow-through if needed
W/C Mobility	X			To enable her to be independent in various aspects of school activities
Transfers	X			Same as above
Functional Ambulation	X			Same as above
Functional Communication			X	Area not affected by current diagnosis
Object Manipulation			X	Same as above
Psychological/Emotional Daily Living Skills				
Self-Concept/Self-Identity	X			To assist with adjustment to an environment with children who are not physically impaired
Situational Coping	X			Same as above
Community Involvement	X			Same as above
Work				
Homemaking		X		Assist parents in assigning appropriate household chores to enhance family role
Child Care/Parenting			X	
Employment Preparation			X	
Play/Leisure	X			Identify limitations and capabilities to held guide students and teachers in appropriate activities

Evaluation Checklist

Patient Name: Patient D

LEGEND: R—RELEVANT; SR—SOMEWHAT RELEVANT; N/A—NOT APPLICABLE

Category	Rating R	Rating SR	Rating N/A	Comments
B. Sensorimotor Components				
Neuromuscular				
Reflex Integration	X			Identifies limitations for school activities
Range of Motion	X			Relevant to diagnosis specifically in lower extremities
PROM	X			Same as above
AROM	X			Same as above
A/AROM	X			Same as above
Gross and Fine Coordination				
Muscle Control		X		To ensure skills are developing appropriately
Coordination		X		Same as above
Dexterity		X		Same as above
Strength and Endurance	X			Specifically upper-body strength secondary to diagnosis
Sensory Integration			X	
Sensory Awareness	X			Lower extremity sensory testing
Visual-Spatial Awareness			X	Not relevant to diagnosis
Body Integration				
Body Schema	X			Relevant per diagnosis
Postural Balance	X			Same as above
(B) Motor Coordination		X		Ensure appropriate development for her age
Right-Left Discrimination		X		Same as above
Visual-Motor Integration		X		Same as above
Crossing Midline			X	Area not affected by diagnosis
Praxis			X	Same as above
C. Cognitive Components				
Orientation		X		Areas not affected by diagnosis, but could be developmentally delayed secondary to past environment

Evaluation Checklist continued

Patient Name: Patient D

LEGEND: R—RELEVANT; SR—SOMEWHAT RELEVANT; N/A—NOT APPLICABLE

Category	Rating			Comments
	R	SR	N/A	
Conceptualization/Comprehension		X		Areas not affected by diagnosis, but could be developmentally delayed secondary to past environment
Concentration		X		Same as above
Attention Span		X		Same as above
Memory		X		Same as above
Cognitive Integration				
Generalizing		X		Areas not affected by diagnosis, but could be developmentally delayed secondary to past environment
Problem Solving		X		Same as above
Defining or Evaluating a Problem		X		Same as above
Organizing a Plan		X		Same as above
Implementing a Plan		X		Same as above
Evaluating a Decision		X		Same as above
D. Psychosocial Components				
Self-Management				
Self-Expression		X		Area not affected by diagnosis, but could be developmentally delayed secondary to environment
Self-Control		X		Same as above
Dyadic Interaction		X		Same as above
Group Interaction		X		Same as above
E. Therapeutic Adaptations				
Orthotics		X		Possible for lower extremities or trunk during ambulation
Prosthetics			X	Not relevant to diagnosis
Assistive/Adaptive Equipment	X			To compensate for decreased lower extremity functioning for mobility and/or self-care
F. Prevention				
Energy Conservation		X		To assist with transitioning to a full day of classes and activities

Evaluation Checklist continued

Patient Name: Patient D

LEGEND: R—RELEVANT; SR—SOMEWHAT RELEVANT; N/A—NOT APPLICABLE

Category	Rating			Comments
	R	SR	N/A	
Joint Protection/Body Mechanics	X			Maintain lower extremity and trunk joint and muscle integrity
Positioning	X			Same as above
Coordination of Daily Living Activities	X			Organize ADL due to new environment and expectations with her specific limitations

Evaluation Checklist continued

Patient Name: Patient D

LEGEND: R—RELEVANT; SR—SOMEWHAT RELEVANT; N/A—NOT APPLICABLE

Evaluation chart adapted from the *Reference Manual of the Official Documents of the American Occupational Therapy Association, Inc.* (pp. VIII.22–23) by The American Occupational Therapy Association, 1986, Rockville, MD: Author.

Exercise 1:2—Patient E

A) Diagnosis:

THR

- Look up as total hip arthroplasty: Surgical replacement of head and neck of the femur. Process that cements a self-curing acrylic resin to adhere a plastic acetabular cup to the pelvis and a metal prosthetic femoral head to the hollowed-out femur.
- Postoperative precautions (posterior approach): Avoid hip flexion past 70°–80° for first 2 months to allow soft tissue to heal after surgery. No passive range of motion of hip. Ambulation promoted quickly (full weight bearing). ADL training to maintain hip precautions.

B) Phase of recovery:

- Acute because of precautions.

C) Facility considerations:

- Patient seen 30 minutes each day for 2 weeks.

D) Other significant areas:

- Patient lives in a nursing home and discharge plans are to return to the nursing home.
- Severe RA: A systemic disease characterized by remissions and exacerbations that vary in severity and timing among people. Symptoms involve pain, stiffness, and limited movement in joints, malaise, fatigue, wasting of muscles around joints, and anemia. After an exacerbation, joints are left progressively deformed. Treatment approach is prevention of joint deformity and pain for as long as possible. Excess joint play is due to loosened ligaments and joint capsules, and contracture of muscles and other connective tissue.

Reference: Trombly, C.A. (1989). Occupational therapy for physical dysfunction (3rd ed.). Baltimore: Williams & Wilkins.

See the following Evaluation Checklist for Patient E.

Category	Rating R	SR	N/A	Comments
A. Independent Living/Daily Living Skills				
Physical Daily Living Skills				
Grooming and Hygiene		X		Simple self-care tasks, but most will be provided to maintain precautions
Feeding/Eating		X		Same as above
Dressing		X		Same as above
Functional Mobility				
Bed Mobility	X			To maintain skin integrity and decrease need for nursing staff in nursing home
W/C Mobility		X		
Transfers	X			Skill that is needed in nursing home
Functional Ambulation	X			Same as above
Functional Communication			X	Not affected by diagnosis or history
Object Manipulation		X		Hands nonfunctional prior to this diagnosis, but may be able to provide adaptations
Psychological/Emotional Daily Living Skills				
Self-Concept/Self-Identity		X		
Situational Coping	X			
Community Involvement			X	Time does not allow to evaluate
Work				
Homemaking			X	Not applicable according to discharge plans
Child Care/Parenting			X	Same as above
Employment Preparation			X	Same as above
Play/Leisure		X		Evaluate to enable patient to participate in nursing home activities

Evaluation Checklist

Patient Name: Patient E

LEGEND: R—RELEVANT; SR—SOMEWHAT RELEVANT; N/A—NOT APPLICABLE

Category	Rating			Comments
	R	SR	N/A	
B. Sensorimotor Components				
Neuromuscular				
Reflex Integration			X	Not applicable for current or past diagnosis
Range of Motion				
PROM	X			Determine current status
AROM	X			Same as above
A/AROM	X			Same as above
Gross and Fine Coordination				
Muscle Control	X			Determine current status
Coordination		X		Same as above
Dexterity		X		Same as above
Strength and Endurance		X		Formal strength test deferred secondary to joint integrity per diagnosis. Endurance to compensate for RA effects
Sensory Integration			X	Not related to diagnosis (past or present)
Sensory Awareness			X	Same as above
Visual-Spatial Awareness			X	Same as above
Body Integration				
Body Schema			X	Not related to diagnosis (past or present)
Postural Balance	X			Will be affected secondary to total hip replacement
(B) Motor Coordination		X		Use of upper extremities to assist with ambulation
Right-Left Discrimination			X	Not related to diagnosis (past or present)
Visual-Motor Integration			X	Same as above
Crossing Midline			X	Same as above
Praxis			X	Same as above
C. Cognitive Components				
Orientation		X		To determine any complications with surgery and pt's current status

Evaluation Checklist continued

Patient Name: Patient E

LEGEND: R—RELEVANT; SR—SOMEWHAT RELEVANT; N/A—NOT APPLICABLE

Category	Rating R	SR	N/A	Comments
Conceptualization/Comprehension	X			To determine if patient can maintain THR precautions
Concentration		X		Same as above
Attention Span		X		Same as above
Memory	X			Same as above
Cognitive Integration				
Generalizing		X		To determine if patient can maintain THR precautions
Problem Solving		X		Same as above
Defining or Evaluating a Problem			X	Not related to diagnosis (past or present) or discharge planning
Organizing a Plan			X	Same as above
Implementing a Plan			X	Same as above
Evaluating a Decision			X	Same as above
D. Psychosocial Components				
Self-Management				
Self-Expression			X	
Self-Control			X	Not related to diagnosis (past or present)
Dyadic Interaction			X	
Group Interaction			X	
E. Therapeutic Adaptations				
Orthotics		X		May be needed for positioning hands secondary to arthritis
Prosthetics			X	Not related to diagnosis (past or present)
Assistive/Adaptive Equipment		X		May be needed to assist with bed or chair positioning to maintain precautions
F. Prevention				
Energy Conservation			X	Not needed secondary to nursing home placement
Joint Protection/Body Mechanics	X			Evaluate for arthritic condition
Positioning	X			Evaluate for both THR precautions and arthritis
Coordination of Daily Living Activities			X	Not relevant secondary to nursing home placement

Evaluation Checklist continued

Patient Name: Patient E

LEGEND: R—RELEVANT; SR—SOMEWHAT RELEVANT; N/A—NOT APPLICABLE

Evaluation chart adapted from the *Reference Manual of the Official Documents of the American Occupational Therapy Association, Inc.* (pp. VIII.22–23) by The American Occupational Therapy Association, 1986, Rockville, MD: Author.

Exercise 1:2—Patient F

A) Diagnosis:

CVA, occlusion of the internal carotid artery

- Occlusion can be caused by thrombosis or embolism.
- Can produce contralateral signs: Homonymous hemianopsia, central type of facial paralysis, hemiparesis or hemiplegia, hemisensory loss, dysphagia, aphasia.
- Acute phase usually causes impairment of consciousness (drowsiness to coma).

Reference: Gilroy, J., & Holliday, P.L. (1982). *Basic neurology.* New York: Macmillan.

B) Phase of recovery:

- Acute; patient is medically unstable.

C) Facility considerations:

- ICU environment limits therapy sessions to short periods due to medical needs and patient's medical status.

D) Other significant areas:

- Past medical history: MI and IDDM.
- Future placement plans: Transfer to acute care and then to rehab unit.
- Patient's functional level prior to incident.

See the following Evaluation Checklist for Patient F.

Category	Rating R	Rating SR	Rating N/A	Comments
A. Independent Living/Daily Living Skills				
Physical Daily Living Skills				
Grooming and Hygiene		X		Simple grooming tasks may be evaluated
Feeding/Eating		X		May be appropriate if the patient is able to eat
Dressing			X	Patient's endurance level and medical status not appropriate
Functional Mobility				
Bed Mobility	X			Enable patient to be functional and maintain skin integrity
W/C Mobility			X	Patient unable to tolerate at this time
Transfers		X		May be appropriate for sitting in chair by bed
Functional Ambulation			X	Patient unable to tolerate at this time
Functional Communication	X			Diagnosis and endurance level appropriate
Object Manipulation	X			Same as above
Psychological/Emotional Daily Living Skills				
Self-Concept/Self-Identity		X		Can assist in determining cognitive status
Situational Coping	X			
Community Involvement			X	Patient's medical status interferes with this activity
Work				
Homemaking			X	Patient's medical status interferes with this activity
Child Care/Parenting			X	Same as above
Employment Preparation			X	Same as above
Play/Leisure			X	Same as above

Evaluation Checklist

Patient Name: Patient F

LEGEND: R—RELEVANT; SR—SOMEWHAT RELEVANT; N/A—NOT APPLICABLE

Category	Rating			Comments
	R	SR	N/A	
B. Sensorimotor Components				
Neuromuscular				
Reflex Integration	X			Diagnosis and endurance level appropriate
Range of Motion				
PROM	X			Diagnosis and endurance level appropriate
AROM	X			Same as above
A/AROM	X			Same as above
Gross and Fine Coordination				
Muscle Control	X			Diagnosis and endurance level appropriate
Coordination	X			Same as above
Dexterity	X			Same as above
Strength and Endurance	X			Same as above
Sensory Integration		X		Same as above
Sensory Awareness	X			Diagnosis and endurance level appropriate for brief evaluation
Visual-Spatial Awareness	X			Same as above
Body Integration				
Body Schema	X			Diagnosis and endurance level appropriate for brief evaluation
Postural Balance		X		Appropriate if patient is able to sit up
(B) Motor Coordination		X		Impaired by diagnosis; determines level of impairment
Right-Left Discrimination	X			Same as above
Visual-Motor Integration	X			Same as above
Crossing Midline	X			Same as above
Praxis	X			Same as above
C. Cognitive Components				
Orientation	X			Impaired by diagnosis; determines level of impairment
Conceptualization/Comprehension	X			Same as above

Evaluation Checklist continued

Patient Name: Patient F

LEGEND: R—RELEVANT; SR—SOMEWHAT RELEVANT; N/A—NOT APPLICABLE

Category	Rating			Comments
	R	SR	N/A	
Concentration	X			Impaired by diagnosis; determines level of impairment
Attention Span	X			Same as above
Memory	X			Same as above
Cognitive Integration				
Generalizing			X	Task too complicated for level of functioning
Problem Solving			X	Same as above
Defining or Evaluating a Problem			X	Same as above
Organizing a Plan			X	Same as above
Implementing a Plan			X	Same as above
Evaluating a Decision			X	Same as above
D. Psychosocial Components				
Self-Management				
Self-Expression		X		Related to dx and appropriate for endurance
Self-Control		X		Same as above
Dyadic Interaction		X		Same as above
Group Interaction			X	N/A for current situation
E. Therapeutic Adaptations				
Orthotics	X			Possible splints for hands and/or feet
Prosthetics			X	N/A for diagnosis
Assistive/Adaptive Equipment	X			Possible for bed positioning
F. Prevention				
Energy Conservation			X	N/A for current medical status
Joint Protection/Body Mechanics	X			For UE and LE positioning
Positioning	X			Appropriate bed positioning
Coordination of Daily Living Activities			X	N/A for current medical status

Evaluation Checklist continued

Patient Name: Patient F

LEGEND: R—RELEVANT; SR—SOMEWHAT RELEVANT; N/A—NOT APPLICABLE

Evaluation chart adapted from the *Reference Manual of the Official Documents of the American Occupational Therapy Association, Inc.* (pp. VIII.22–23) by The American Occupational Therapy Association, 1986, Rockville, MD: Author.

Exercise 1:3a—Margaret

A) Medications:

- Percocet N100 p.r.n.: Analgesic and sedative, relief of mild to moderately severe pain. Possible side effects: lightheadedness, dizziness, sedation, nausea, vomiting.
- Aspirin (acetylsalicylic acid): Antiinflammatory analgesic, treatment of arthritis. Possible side effects: Stomach distress, heartburn, peptic ulcers.
- Heparin: Anticoagulant, anticoagulant therapy in prophylaxis and treatment of venous thrombosis, prevention of postoperative deep vein thrombosis, prevention and treatment of peripheral arterial embolism. Possible side effects: Hemorrhage, local irritation, chills, fever, urticaria.

B) Interview information:

- Does she live alone?
- Physical set-up of home (e.g., stairs)
- Routine activity in a day. Daily responsibilities.
- Is anyone available to assist her for a few weeks?
- How does she feel now, and what is her opinion of going home in a week?

C) Physical status information:

- Upper extremity range of motion and strength: Will need to use upper extremities to compensate for decreased ability to use lower extremities during recovery and to maintain hip precautions for teaching, dressing body skills.
- Transfer status (chairs, bed, commode), car transfers, and shower transfers: For safety and function.
- Bed mobility: To maintain skin integrity and to facilitate function.
- Functional ambulation: For safe household mobility.
- Postural balance: For safety during functional activities.

D) Cognitive status information:

- Comprehension, concentration, attention, memory, generalization, problem resolution, plan organization: To ensure patient will be able to maintain THR precautions during functional activities.

E) Patient evaluation information:

- Need to identify Margaret's mode and endurance level for ambulation status, including her endurance, the equipment she uses, and how much assistance she requires.

F) Areas to be addressed:

- Hygiene
- Bed mobility
- Grooming
- Functional transfers
- Dressing
- Household mobility

Exercise 1:3b—Beulah

A) Medications:

- Parlodel: Dopamine receptor agonist, treatment of signs and symptoms of idiopathic or postencephalitic Parkinson's disease. Possible side effects: Nausea, headache, dizziness, fatigue.
- Macrodantin: Antibacterial, treatment of urinary tract infection. Possible side effects: Pulmonary hypersensitivity, malaise, dyspnea on exertion, cough, nausea, emesis.
- Tylenol® #3 p.r.n.: Centrally acting analgesic (codeine) and peripherally acting analgesic (acetaminophen), for relief of mild to moderately severe pain due to surgery. Possible side effects: Lightheadedness, dizziness, sedation, shortness of breath, nausea, vomiting.

B) Patient is oriented to person but not to place. She is confused and is unreliable for current personal history information.

C) Beulah may have Parkinson's dementia or may still be suffering from the side effects of the surgical anesthetic.

D) Social service:

- Her previous functional level, including self-care skills, household mobility, and cognitive status.
- Level of care she required prior to current hospitalization. (Was she left alone? Did she need physical assistance for activities of daily living?)
- Current support system (i.e., friends, family).

E) Yes.

- Activities to increase and maintain joint range of motion, strength, and coordination as a result of the Parkinson's process.
- Functional mobility, transfers, and bed mobility. (Improving these areas will help Beulah's caregivers take care of her safely.)
- Family education for her caregivers to assist them with providing care.
- Not dressing or bathing skills because Beulah's cognitive status would interfere with her ability to perform the tasks safely and consistently.

Exercise 1:3c—Tom

A) Medications:

- Heparin: Anticoagulant to maintain patency of an indwelling venipuncture device designed for intermittent injections, infusion therapy, or blood sampling (IV). Possible side effects: Hemorrhage, local irritation, chills, fever, urticaria.
- Procardia: Antianginal for management of vasospastic angina. Possible side effects: Dizziness, lightheadedness, giddiness, flushing, heat sensation.
- Insulin and humulin insulin NPH: Regular insulin with an intermediate-acting insulin, treatment of diabetes mellitus. Possible side effects: Sweating, dizziness, palpitations, tremors, hunger.

B) Ask questions related to orientation, memory, attention span, concentration, and comprehension.

C) Right upper extremity:

- Sensation
- Reflex integration
- Active/passive range of motion (joint integrity)
- Muscle control (tone)
- Coordination/dexterity

To determine if current diagnosis had any bilateral effect. Provides a baseline of information that may be used to relate to the patient's prior functional level.

D) Left upper extremity:

- Sensation
- Reflex integration
- Active/passive range of motion (joint integrity)
- Muscle control (tone)
- Coordination/dexterity

To determine baseline of information. Right cerebrovascular accident commonly shows neurological effects on left side of body.

E) Ask questions related to the patient's visual area.

F) Perform manual muscle tests in gravity; eliminate positions and provide various types of facilitation techniques to activate muscle contractions.

Exercise 1:3d—Ed

A) Medications:

- Coumadin: Anticoagulant, prophylaxis and/or treatment of venous thrombosis. Possible side effects: Hemorrhage, necrosis of skin, alopecia, urticaria, dermatitis.
- Verapamil hydrochloride: Calcium influx inhibitor, management of essential hypertension. Possible side effects: Diarrhea, dry mouth, ecchymosis, confusion, muscle cramps, blurred vision.

B) Hemianopsia, visual neglect, or embarrassment. Engage Ed in purposeful activities and observe his ability to look to the left. Perform a standardized test to evaluate his visual field integrity.

C) Rehabilitative services:

- Speech therapy to address communication deficits.
- Social Services to evaluate home situation and patient's functional status prior to his cerebrovascular accident.
- Physical therapy to execute an ambulation evaluation.

D) Social services and possibly nursing staff.

Social Services' evaluation includes history from family on the patient's current living situation and personality traits. Nursing may have had direct contact with the family.

E) Gross motor skills (e.g., through bed mobility, transfers) and upper extremity status. Further evaluation on cognitive skills or communication should probably be avoided until rapport has been developed.

The answer on technique depends on the areas selected and the student's choice of evaluation tools.

Exercise 1:3e—Warren

A) Medications:

- Humulin insulin NPH: Human insulin isophane suspension, management of diabetes. Possible side effects: Sweating, dizziness, palpitations, tremors, hunger.
- Inderal: Beta-adrenergic receptor blocking agent, long-term management of cardiac arrhythmias. Possible side effects: Bradycardia, arterial insufficiency, lightheadedness, depression.
- Tylenol® #3 p.r.n.: Centrally acting analgesic (codeine) and peripherally acting analgesic (acetaminophen), for relief of mild to moderately severe pain, phantom pain of amputated stump. Possible side effects: Lightheadedness, dizziness, sedation, shortness of breath, nausea, vomiting.

B) Phantom pain or sensation. Provide various types of desensitization techniques and encourage use of his prosthesis.

C) Areas to evaluate:

- Grooming/hygiene
- Postural balance
- Dressing
- Orientation
- Bed mobility
- Comprehension
- Wheelchair mobility
- Concentration
- Transfers
- Attention span
- Functional mobility
- Memory
- Situational coping
- Cognitive integration skills
- Self-concept
- Positioning of stump
- Active and passive ranges of motion of upper extremities
- Stump edema
- Sensory awareness

All of these functional areas may be affected secondary to the diagnosis. The patient will need these skills in order to return to functional independence.

D) Activities to increase prosthetic tolerance while weight bearing or weight shifting. After each treatment, check stump for pressure areas.

E) Yes, to prepare for times when prosthesis is not worn. For example, if stump develops complications at night, or if prosthesis requires repair.

F) Three areas of focus:
   - Functional ambulation
   - Functional transfers
   - Activities of daily living with and without prosthesis

Exercise 1:3f—Sara

A) Areas to evaluate:

- Active range of motion, passive range of motion, and strength of right upper extremity
- Active range of motion, passive range of motion, and strength of residual joints of left upper extremity
- Muscle control of left upper extremity
- Sensory status of left upper extremity and stump area
- Cognitive status and functioning
- Situational coping
- Self-concept/self-identity
- Stump condition (edema, pattern of healing)

B) Social Services and/or Case Management

- If the patient and the family would be in favor of a prosthesis and if equipment is covered by insurance
- If there would be a need to identify an alternative method of payment.

C) One-handed self-care skills. Maintain or regain strength and range of motion in upper extremities. Control edema and assist with appropriate stump shaping. Reduce or prevent phantom limb phenomenon. Approach to the physician should include these areas in order to justify continued treatment.

Exercise 1:3g—Phillip

A) Head rest, head blocks, reclining wheelchair, lap trays or some type of upper extremity support devices, seat cushion, solid seat, elevating leg rests, lateral supports to stabilize trunk, seat belt or posey support.

B) Nursing can provide information about skin integrity that can be used for effective positioning.

C) Evaluation with physical therapy:

- Bed mobility
- Endurance for activity
- Transfers
- Postural balance
- Reflex integration
- Positioning
- Passive/active range of motion
- Assistive/adaptive equipment related to positioning
- Muscle tone
- Situational coping
- Sensory awareness
- Sensory integration

D) Evaluation with speech therapist:

- Functional communication
- Self-expression
- Feeding/eating
- Self-control
- Situational coping
- Visual-spatial awareness
- Orientation
- Comprehension
- Concentration
- Attention span

Exercise 1:3h—Nancy

A) Medications:

- Nonsteroidal antiinflammatory (NSAID): Control of arthritis pain. Possible side effects: None.
- Prednisone: Glucocortoid steroid, for short-term management of acute exacerbation of RA. Possible side effects: Muscle weakness; steroid myopathy may suppress reactions to skin tests. Caution not to overstress joints for ROM and strength testing because pain is masked.

B) Most information needs to be gathered during the interview process secondary to outpatient status. The information is used to determine Nancy's current level of functioning and to plan educational intervention.

- Grooming/hygiene
- Feeding/eating
- Dressing
- Object manipulation
- Situational coping
- Child care/homemaking
- Play/leisure
- Active/passive range of motion
- Joint integrity
- Muscle control
- Endurance
- Strength (if no joint deformities and joints not inflamed, not at (L) shoulder secondary to Prednisone injection)
- Energy conservation
- Joint protection/body mechanics
- Positioning
- Prosthetics

C) Yes, use positioning splints.

D) Approach to physician should include an explanation that the splints maintain joint alignment which, in turn, prevents pain and joint deformities.

Exercise 1:3i—Timothy

A) Medications:

- Colace: Stool softener, to ease stool passage due to C-5–C-6 spinal cord injury. Possible side effects: Nausea, rash.
- Metamucil/Dulcolax: Natural therapeutic fiber to manage constipation; combined Colace, Metamucil, and Dulcolax for a bowel and bladder program. Possible side effects: Possible abdominal discomfort.
- Valium: Induces calming effects to decrease spasticity caused by upper motor neuron disorders. Possible side effects: Drowsiness, fatigue, and ataxia upon abrupt withdrawal; convulsions; tremors.

B) Evaluate:

- Bed mobility
- Functional communication
- Conceptualization/concentration
- Object manipulation
- Attention span
- Self-concept/self-identity
- Memory
- Orthotics
- Reflex integration
- Adaptive equipment (for positioning)
- Active/passive range of motion
- Joint protection
- Muscle control
- Positioning
- Sensory awareness
- Visual-spatial awareness
- Postural balance
- Orientation
- Situational coping

All of these functional areas may be affected secondary to the diagnosis. The patient will need these skills in order to return to functional independence.

C) Yes, physical therapy.

Evaluate:

- Bed mobility
- Orthotics
- Reflex integration
- Adaptive equipment (for positioning)
- Active/passive range of motion
- Joint protection
- Muscle control

- Positioning
- Sensory awareness
- Visual-spatial awareness
- Postural balance
- Orientation

D) Precautions related to sympathetic hyperreflexion or autonomic dysreflexia. The autonomic nervous system is likely to be affected secondary to diagnosis.

Exercise 1:3j—Mary

A) Medications:

- Nimodipine (for 21 days): Inhibits contraction of vascular smooth muscle, improves of neurological outcome by reducing the incidence and severity of ischemic deficits in patients with subarachnoid hemorrhage from ruptured congenital aneurysms. Possible side effects: Edema, rash.
- Heparin: Anticoagulant, for anticoagulant therapy in prophylaxis for venous thrombosis. Possible side effects: Hemorrhage, local irritation, chills, fever, urticaria.

B) Disturbance of cerebellum functioning can produce:

- Ataxia
- Intension tremor
- Nystagmus
- Dysmetria (disturbed ability to gauge distances)
- Dysdiadochokinesia (disturbed ability to perform rapid alternating movements)
- Hypotonia and rebound

Reference: Gilroy, J., & Holliday, P.L. (1982). *Basic neurology*. New York: Macmillan.

Disturbances of left temporal lobe region for most individuals who are right-hand dominant can produce:

- Receptive aphasia
- Wernicke's area disturbances
- Spatial relation disturbances
- Disturbances in the auditory cortex

Reference: Guyton, A.C. (1981). *Textbook of medical physiology*. Philadelphia: W.B. Saunders.

Disturbances can be related to motor control functioning secondary to cerebellum damage or cognitive deficits secondary to temporal lobe damage.

C) Evaluate Mary by isolating cognitive instruction and UE control activities to determine the true deficit areas in the following ways:

- Have Mary imitate arm movements with physical cues only (evaluates motor control).
- Have Mary do a repetitive task after you demonstrate it and only use physical cues. Try one hand at a time and then try bilateral tasks (evaluates motor control).
- Give Mary a spontaneous motor activity. For example, fold a towel and then give her one to fold.
- Ask Mary to do simple body commands. Start with the facial area and work down, because cranial nerves may not be affected. For example, stick out tongue or blink eyes.
- Ask Mary to identify objects by looking at them. For example, have her find the stove or the refrigerator.
- Evaluate Mary's ability to respond to gestures or written information.

D) Evaluate:

- Grooming/hygiene
- Feeding/eating
- Dressing
- Bed mobility
- Transfers
- Situational coping
- Neuromuscular status
- Reflex integration
- Active/passive range of motion
- Body integration components
- Cognitive components
- Positioning joint protection

All of these functional areas may be affected secondary to the diagnosis. The patient will need these skills in order to return to functional independence.

Exercise 2:1b—Carol

D)

1. **Strengths:**

- Carol has equipment that can assist her at home.
- Her upper extremity strength, skin condition, and active range of motion are assets.
- She appears motivated to assist her mother as much as she can with her self-care.

Weaknesses:

- Functional transfer status could change secondary to prognosis of left foot/ankle.
- Upper extremity sensation is impaired bilaterally.
- Decreased visual status
- Deteriorating health, which interferes with the relationship with her mother.
- Decreased gross mobility skills (sit to supine)

2.

- Increased upper extremity strength to compensate for her possible loss of lower extremity functioning.
- Increased ability to compensate for her decreased vision with ADL exercises to improve independence.
- Improved gross motor skills (through training)
- Ways to stimulate a positive relationship between her and her mother.

3.

- Increase bilateral upper extremity strength to good.
- Carol will be able to dress herself with minimal assistance.
- Carol will be independent for bed mobility (sit to supine).
- Carol and her mother will identify two leisure activities they can share.

4. Activities should relate to increasing upper extremity strength, self-care, bed mobility, and leisure skill identification.

Exercise 2:1c—Kevin

D)

1. **Strengths:**

- Upper extremity strength and range of motion status
- Cognitive status
- Age
- Basic ADL status
- Motivation for appropriate independent living skills

Weaknesses:

- Community functional transfers
- Community wheelchair mobility
- Dynamic sitting balance
- Equipment issued not appropriate to maximize independence (e.g., standard wheelchair)
- The relationship that Kevin has with his parents appears to foster his dependence.

2.

- Increased community mobility.
- Increased functional transfers.
- Increased general independence and self-confidence to allow Kevin's relationship with his parents to develop toward his goals.
- Situational coping skills that will assist Kevin with his transition back to school and his role in the relationship with his girlfriend.

3.

- Evaluate Kevin for a lightweight wheelchair to increase his independence with the equipment.
- Increase Kevin's ability to perform wheelchair mobility on various surface grades and in community settings.
- Teach Kevin advanced transfer skills to include floor transfers, community bathroom transfers, and car transfers.
- Assist Kevin in identifying leisure interest skills or hobbies and teach relaxation methods.

4. Activities should relate to community wheelchair mobility, advanced transfers, relaxation techniques, and leisure skill development.

Exercise 2:1d—Ethel

D)

1. **Strengths:**

- Cognitive status
- General mobility
- Motivation to return home as independent as possible

Weaknesses:

- Decreased weight bearing on left lower extremity secondary to pain
- Hand functioning
- Decreased functional mobility
- Lack of assistive equipment for home use
- Decreased ADL skills secondary to hip precautions

2.

- She will need to be independent with dressing and maintaining her THR precautions.
- She will need to be independent in household mobility.
- She will need to maintain THR precautions during bathing and dressing, which will require equipment to assist her.

3.

- Dressing and bathing lower extremities.
- Household mobility skills using the walker.
- Train her to use equipment (e.g., tub bench, long-handled sponge, sock aid, long-handled shoe horn) safely.

4. Activities should relate to dressing, bathing training, household mobility, and adaptive equipment training.

Exercise 2:1e—Schoci

D)

1. **Strengths:**

- Supportive family with traditional views
- Left upper extremity functioning (generally)
- Head and postural control

Weaknesses:

- Orientation
- Right upper extremity status
- Left upper extremity strength
- Transfer status
- Sitting balance
- Bed mobility
- Perception
- Self-care status
- Communication

2.

- Extensive home care techniques. Complete independence of skills not desired because of the traditional beliefs of the family.
- Safe transfer and bed mobility techniques.
- Increased Schoci's left upper extremity strength and sitting balance to enhance the family's ability to care for Schoci.

3.

- Increase transfer ability at least to a level where one person can perform the transfers safely.
- Increase bed mobility to independent. Allows patient to perform weight shifting in bed so family does not need to monitor her every 2 hours. Mobility also assists family members during care routines.
- Increase sitting balance for the patient's safety and to assist the family with general care.
- Provide technique training for bathing, dressing, transfers, left upper extremity care, and mobility to protect family members who are providing care from injury.
- Increase left upper extremity strength to enable Schoci to assist with her self-care without interfering with the family's traditional beliefs.

4. Activities should relate to increasing transferring ability, bed mobility skills, sitting balance, family training, and left upper extremity strengthening without an emphasis on self-care independence.

Exercise 2:1e—Schoci (continued)

D)

1. **Strengths:**

- Schoci's desire to return to functional independence and her family's support
- Left upper extremity functioning (generally)
- Head and postural control

Weaknesses:

- Orientation
- Right upper extremity status
- Left upper extremity strength
- Transfer status
- Sitting balance
- Bed mobility
- Perception
- Self-care status
- Communication

2.

- Become oriented to her environment.
- Increase right upper extremity functioning and/or learn to protect the arm.
- Increase transferring ability in order to be as independent as possible.
- Show good compensation for perception deficits to increase safety.
- Be able to perform activities of daily living as independently as possible.
- Have a safe mode of functional mobility.
- Know one-handed techniques for activities of daily living and independent living skills.

3.

- Schoci will need to be oriented to time and place in order to become functionally independent.
- Provide support for right upper extremity to prevent further subluxation or pain and facilitate functioning for arm.
- She will need to increase her ability to weight bear on her left lower extremity or increase general endurance and balance to improve transfers.
- She will need to improve her dynamic sitting balance strength to assist with transfers and general mobility.
- She will need to become aware of her right visual deficits and learn compensation techniques.
- She will need to be able to dress and bathe herself, and perform hygiene and grooming needs as independently as possible.
- She will need to work on lower extremity weight bearing, sitting balance, and visual compensation to lead to functional ambulation or wheelchair mobility.
- Possible equipment needs: Arm trough/lap tray to support left upper extremity, wheelchair, tub transfer bench, one-handed appliances.

- Teach one-handed techniques for household functioning.

4. Activities should relate to increasing orientation, right upper extremity functioning, left lower extremity weight bearing, postural balance, dynamic sitting balance, education/compensation techniques for visual neglect, dressing and hygiene training, and adaptive equipment training.

Exercise 2:1f—Extra Credit

D) Provide training to the nursing aides regarding the purpose and rationale for occupational therapy. Also, provide training on how to monitor skin conditions and splint applications. Provide rationale for splint use.

Develop a splint-wearing schedule that can be used facility-wide and a recreation calendar. Give an inservice to educate the staff on the use of the schedule and calendar.

Develop a method to notify physicians of the new services that will be offered. Also, inform physicians that they will need to provide a referral for services (e.g., memo to all consulting physicians). Include a description of a documentation process.

Develop a documentation system by consulting administration, appropriate regulations based on the primary pay sources, and the medical director.

Exercise 2:2a—Debbie

A) Planes or patterns of shoulder movement described in the picture are horizontal shoulder abduction and adduction.

B) There are two points of view for using muscle grading. One view considers using muscle grades as inappropriate for any neurological patient because of the muscle tone influence caused by the central nervous system damage. Another view considers using the muscle grading system if the muscle tone is normal and there is isolated movement in muscles; not synergies. This system is convenient for reporting function.

If a professional chooses to use the muscle grading system, Debbie's shoulder strength would be described as "poor" for shoulder horizontal abduction and adduction. The deltoid aid provides a gravity-eliminated environment, and the arm can move in partial range.

C) Shoulder flexion/extension—side lying on the mat. Internal and external rotation—keep patient in sitting position.

D) Consult techniques developed by the following approaches:

- Rood Approach
- Bobath Neurodevelopmental Approach
- Brunnstrom Approach
- Proprioceptive Neuromuscular Approach (PNF)
- Carr and Shepherd Approach

E) Consult stroke recovery patterns. The natural course of return of motor function is from proximal to distal and from mass, patterned, undifferentiated movement to fine, isolated movement. This indicates there would not be a concentrated effort on active finger or hand movement at this time.

Reference: Trombly, C.A. (1989). *Occupational Therapy for Physical Dysfunction* (3rd ed.) Baltimore: Williams & Wilkins.

F) Use the methods developed for describing the patient's movement and the therapy techniques that have been explored in Section D and formulate them into functional goals using verb, action, and measurable end point.

Exercise 2:2b—Phillip

A) Occupational therapy goals should include verbs, action, and measurable end points. Areas of focus can include:

- Tolerating gross motor movement
- Tolerating splints for hand/joint protection
- Increasing head control to tolerate removal of head rest for short lengths of time
- General tolerance for activity
- Tolerance for being in wheelchair with positioning

B) Wheelchair equipment suggestions:

- Reclining wheelchair/cushion
- Elevating leg rests
- Head rest
- Lap tray or supportive arm troughs
- Lateral supports
- Head blocks
- Seat belt for posey

Tolerance schedule: 2 hours at a time

C) Occupational therapy goals should include verbs, action, and measurable end-points. Areas of focus can include:

- Reliable yes/no responses with eye movements
- Orientation to environment
- Sip-n-puff device for control or head switch
- Tolerate full therapy session

D) The activities should be as functional and age appropriate as possible.

1. Introduce switch devices through remote cars or video games.
2. Ask yes/no response questions in relation to Phillip's interest (e.g., sports, school, girls, cars).
3. Modify games to rely on eye gaze for Phillip to indicate moves or decisions. This method increases eye control, wheelchair tolerance, and head control.

E) Explanation can include:

- "Phillip, your body is not doing what you are telling it to do."
- "This is a very hard time for you, but you are not alone."
- "We need to learn about how to move you and talk to you so you are not scared."
- "You need to learn to talk again."
- "You need to learn to move yourself or walk again."

Be careful; do not create false hopes.

Exercise 2:2c—Cooking group

A) Special diets and feeding precautions such as:

- Diabetic patients
- Restricted sodium, calorie, or cholesterol diets
- Each patient's ability to orally handle food textures (e.g., requires thickened liquid or pureed food textures)

B) Speech pathology to determine feeding precautions and guidelines. Also, dietary to provide each patient's individual restrictions and assist with menu options.

C) Assigned tasks:

- Prepare chicken breast following directions—Cheryl (provide verbal directions)
- Peel and cut carrots—Warren (standing at center)
- Mash and prepare potatoes —Eleanor
- Cut and mix fruit for salad—Warren cut/Eleanor mix
- Set table—Cheryl
- Clear table—Warren and Eleanor
- Wash dishes—Cheryl
- Table conversation suggestions: Topics related to the weather (orientation), current events

D) Formulate goals for each patient's focus of treatment as they relate to the tasks that they have been assigned, using functional area of focus, action, and measurable end point.

- Cheryl—Patient will demonstrate completing a cooking task following verbal directions only.
- Warren—Patient will demonstrate standing with good bilateral weight shifting for 10 minutes.
- Eleanor—Patient will use active range of motion for bilateral upper extremities to perform functional activity with verbal cues.

Exercise 2:2d—Stella (Part 1)

A) Focus of treatment for Stella can include:

- Increasing her sitting balance
- Increasing standing balance
- Teaching self-range of motion for right upper extremity
- Providing activities of daily living training
- Providing family education for right upper extremity care, home evaluation information to modify for safety, and activities of daily living training including tub transfers

B) Outpatient occupational therapy services to provide right upper extremity muscle reeducation, functional ambulation, and increased sitting and standing balance.

C) Formulate functional goals using verb, functional area of focus, and measurable end point based on therapy plan information in Section A. Answers should be based on family education and safety to ensure a comfortable transition to home with the family as the primary caregivers.

Exercise 2:2d—Stella (Part 2)

A) Focus of therapy for Stella can include:

- Increasing sitting balance
- Increasing standing balance
- Teaching muscle facilitation techniques for right upper extremity
- Activities of daily living training
- Tub transfer training
- Household mobility training

B) Formulate functional goals using verb, functional area of focus, and measurable end point based on treatment plan information in Section A. Answers can focus on more developmental recovery strategies because Stella is able to participate in an intensive therapy program.

Exercise 2:2e—Peter

A) Yes. Both therapists addressed right upper extremity functioning and vision perception abilities.

B) No. The activities appropriately addressed Peter's deficits with right upper extremity and vision perception.

C) Sally related the upper extremity activities to Peter's personal goal of wanting to walk. She also explained Peter's visual perception deficits in terms he could understand.

D) No. April's treatment activities did not address Peter's immediate goals and concerns. April did not clearly explain the functional implications of Peter's deficits.

E) This answer varies with each individual's opinion.

F) This answer varies with each individual's opinion.

Exercise 2:2f—Mark (Part 1)

A) Change the position of the pegs on the board to challenge Mark's balance by increasing his reach. For example, reach across his body; reach toward the floor; reach further to his right or left.

B) Relate goal to the functional reaching pattern created by the task in Section A using verb, functional area of focus, and measurable end point.

Exercise 2:2f—Mark (Part 2)

A) Change activity to increase resistance to Mark's left upper extremity. For example, place peg bucket over head to add gravity resistance; add weights.

B) Relate goal to upper extremity strengthening based on the task developed in Section A using verb, functional area of focus, and measurable end point.

Exercise 2:2f—Mark (Part 3)

A) Complete task adding a cognitive component. For example, place pegs in rows by colors; provide a peg design for Mark to copy; give Mark verbal or written activities.

B) Relate goal to Mark's cognitive ability to complete the task provided in Section A using verb, action, and measurable end point.

Exercise 2:2g—Mabel

A) No. The patients with dementia lose the ability to follow directions and rely on spontaneous activities to function. This is a permanent condition.

B) There is a large variety of activities that can be included for each goal. Tasks should be spontaneously functional. Use activity analysis to develop each task.

Exercise 2:2h—Bob

A) Communication should include aspects of:

- Eye contact
- Tone of voice
- Touch
- Facial expression

Examples of communication include statements of reassurance and empathy.

B) Both. Teaching one-handed techniques for function will increase Bob's perception of self-control and independence. Facilitating neurodevelopmental progress for functional recovery of his motor skills will further increase his independence, but it is a slower process.

Exercise 2:2i—Eleanor

A) Visual neglect or hemianopsia.

B) Since you have not completed your evaluation, terms like "sometimes" or "it may be" should be used. Explain how her vision may be damaged.

C) Many possibilities:

- Post a sign that informs visitors of Eleanor's inability to look to the left.
- Change beds with her roommate.
- Inform nursing of the situation.
- Educate Eleanor on the problem and teach her to compensate.

Exercise 2:2j—Dr. Bones

A) Explain the THR procedure in terms that will not insult him. Use a diagram and names of bones. Explain the results of the surgery.

B) Explain the role of occupational therapy in relation to Dr. Bones' diagnosis and his anticipated needs. Include precautions and rationale to achieve functional independence.

Exercise 2:2k—Toni

A) Avoid using terms like edge-of-mat, trunk control, and transfers. Give the parents information on how they can communicate with their daughter. Link the components of the treatment plan to simple functional tasks that are easily understood.

B) May be able to use a few terms to inform Toni's mother about Toni's skills, but explain the terms for her father. Give them information for communication with their daughter. Link the components of the treatment plan to functional abilities that will work toward easing the burden of care.

C) Alternate strengths and weaknesses by monitoring each response of the family. Avoid using terms like "edge-of-mat", "sitting balance", and "receptive aphasia." Explain treatment plan in terms of functional tasks.

Exercise 2:2L—Alan

A) Review the literature for the theoretical causes of phantom pain. Explain the pain to Alan in terms he will understand, considering his education level.

B) Explain the changes in everyday life that Alan will likely experience since his surgery and how occupational therapy will help him prepare for the changes (e.g., bathing, dressing, transfers, walking).

C) Review the literature for the theoretical causes of phantom pain. Explain the pain to Alan considering his age and level of understanding.

Exercise 2:2m—Gerry

A) Answer Gerry's question honestly and reassure him that his mother knows where he is and what he is doing.

B) Answer honestly in terms he can understand. Gerry probably has very little concept of his internal organs and how they affect his health. Explain the role of occupational therapy in terms he can understand.

Exercise 2:2n—Joe

A) Joe could have frontal lobe damage that interferes with his ability to inhibit his behavior. He may be very scared of his current situation or angry. Joe may also feel very vulnerable because of his loss of control over the current situation.

B) Remain very neutral and calm. Explain why you are there and everything you are doing. Explain what you can do for him without giving him false hopes or expectations.

C) Evaluate areas he will be successful in to build his self-confidence. For example, upper extremity control and strength or the interview process.

Exercise 2:2o—Jessica

A) Possible reasons why Jessica's father became angry about the electric wheelchair:

- He may not be able to accept the fact that his daughter will not be able to walk right away.
- Seeing his daughter in a wheelchair may enhance his feelings of helplessness in caring for her.
- He may view the wheelchair as a form of a disability that he had been exposed to in the past and it was not a good experience.

B) Yes. Part of the occupational therapy process includes education that will enable the family to adjust to situations and enhance the quality of the patient's life.

C)

- Do not deny the parents their belief about Jessica's ability to walk again.
- Focus on the fact that walking may take longer to develop than expected, and Jessica's education and social development can continue at a more normal rate while she is undergoing rehabilitation.

D) Do not address the issue with Jessica or in front of her because she should not be confused by the two different opinions. The ultimate decision should be presented to Jessica by her parents.

E) A computer to help her do homework.

Exercise 2:2p—Terri

A)

- Remain calm.
- Introduce yourself.
- Let her know you are here to help her.
- Explain occupational therapy.

B) Review literature for aneurysms. Explain it in terms Terri will understand and explain that she is experiencing the results of the damage caused by the aneurysm bursting.

C) Explain the relationship between the brain functioning and her arm and trunk control.

D) Explain the role of occupational therapy. Explain the evaluation process and what will happen after it is completed.

Exercise 3:1a—Clifford

A) Yes.

B) Outpatient services would provide consistent follow-through with the patient's progress in the rehabilitation program and would be the most cost-effective method of providing services.

C) Therapy plan options for outpatient referral can include:

- Continuing with upper extremity muscle reeducation
- Household mobility training
- Transfer training

D)

- Stroke support group
- Any type of leisure community group

Exercise 3:1b—Bill

A) Yes.

B) Inpatient rehabilitation services would provide a concentrated focus on Bill's recovery. Bill has shown good progress in recovery from the date of onset. It is more cost-effective to continue his recovery progress at this time than to place him in long-term care. Home health would not be able to provide the level of services he needs to make significant gains in independence.

C) Treatment recommendations can include:

- Increased endurance for activity
- Cognitive retraining
- Gross motor skills training
- Upper extremity muscle reeducation for strengthening

D) Community services would not be appropriate for Bill at this time. However, his wife would benefit from any of the following:

- Returning to church participation
- Support group

Exercise 3:1c—Valerie

A) Yes.

B) Outpatient services would be the most beneficial to Valerie and would also be the most cost-effective method to address her rehabilitation needs. Valerie's difficulty with steps will probably not be resolved until she has her cast removed. An outpatient hand clinic would be appropriate because of the complexity of her injuries.

C) The treatment plan could include active range of motion exercises as the patient tolerates. The new therapist would need to contact the physician to progress the program any further.

D) Not many programs would be applicable, due to the fact that Valerie's family is her main support network, and the nature of her injury is temporary.

Exercise 3:1d—Imogene

A) No.

B) Long-term care would be the most appropriate for Imogene due to her level of self-care, her periodic confusion, and the type of support systems she has available. Once her confusion becomes resolved and her THR precautions are removed, Imogene's ability to return home can be reevaluated.

C) Treatment plan options for Imogene's referral may include:

- Follow-up evaluation after THR precautions are removed
- Activities therapy

D) Community programs for Imogene will be addressed at the long-term care facility as they are appropriate. Community programs for the family would probably not be addressed, because the family lives out of town.

Exercise 3:1e—Alice

A) Yes.

B) A reentry program would further increase Alice's self-sufficiency and help her become integrated into vocational and avocational independent living skills.

C) Recommendations could include any level of community independence training and address self-concept and adjustment skills.

D)

- Support group for Alice and her family
- Have Alice or her family contact a recreation facility for adapted sports
- Have Alice or her family contact education administrators at her college

Exercise 3:1f—Homer

A) No. OT services would not be appropriate, but Homer may benefit from a referral to another discipline, such as psychology.

B) None.

C) Family education for his wife so she can provide the level of care he will need at home.

D)

- Contact his previous volunteer employer
- Support group
- Recreation facility that provides consultation for adaptive sports

Exercise 3:2a—Ruth

A) Splint care, application, schedule, and monitoring.

- Joint protection
- Edema control
- Energy conservation

B) Home program:

Name of splint: Volar resting hand splints.

Purpose: To rest involved joints to decrease swelling and pain for RA and to maintain joints in proper alignment.

Schedule: Wear every night.

Directions: Splints should be placed on palm side of hands with the straps attached by matching the numbers.

Splint can be washed with mild soap and water. Do not leave splint in direct sunlight or expose to excessive heat (e.g., in a car during a hot day).

Any excessive pain, lasting red marks (more than 1 hour), excessive swelling, or questions, please call me at ____________________.

Protect your joints.

1. Stop all activities if they produce pain; rest for a while. If pain does not stop in 1 hour, change the way you are doing the activity, using the tips below.
2. Use energy saving devices such as:
   - electric can openers
   - jar openers
   - electric scissors
3. Do not use excessive force, tight grasp, or outward-twisting movements.
   - Use palm to lift heavy objects
   - Twist objects toward thumb side of hand using palm
   - "Palm" pots, pans, coffee cups, buckets; use two hands
4. Control swelling.
   - Elevate hands above heart
   - Do massage from fingertips toward palms, with hands elevated
   - Open and close hands completely throughout the day, while hands are elevated, in order to pump fluids through the body

Exercise 3:2b—Barbara

A) Splint care, application, schedule, and monitoring:
- Exercise program
- Edema control
- Scar massage

B) Home program:

Name of splint: Left volar immobilization splint for 2nd and 3rd digits with wrist in 15°–30° extension, MP in 45° flexion, and slight flexion (15°) of PIP and DIP joints.

Purpose: To prevent overstretching or abrupt movement of fingers while functioning in daily routine.

Schedule: Wear at all times. Remove only for massage and exercises 4 times per day for 15 minute intervals, and hygiene.

Directions: Place splint on the palm side of the left hand with the index and middle fingers in the splint. Attach straps by matching the numbers.

IMPORTANT:

DO exercises at your best times during the day.

DO NOT force any movement past pain.

DO NOT move left hand fingers with right hand.

It is very important that you call me if you have:
- Excessive pain
- Lasting strap marks (more than 1 hour)
- Excessive swelling
- Any questions
- Red areas on skin after removing the splint (lasting more than 15 minutes)

My number is ______________________________.

Splint can be washed with mild soap and water. Do not expose splint to excessive heat (e.g., direct sunlight or in a car during a hot day).

Scar massage: To soften scars, improve movement, and decrease pain:
- Take splint off
- Gently but firmly massage scarred areas with thick ointment, starting at fingertips and working toward wrist, 2 times per day
- Immediately follow with exercises below

Swelling management: To be decreased to prevent permanent stiffness.
- Elevate hand above heart as much as possible
- Move shoulder and elbow in all planes of motion as much as possible
- ake off splint; massage hand with ointment starting at fingertips and stroking toward wrist, make sure arm is elevated—2 times per day
- Immediately follow with the next exercise

Exercise:

1. Hook—Bend only first and second joints (gently), as far as possible, and gently straighten. 5-10 times as tolerated.
2. Straight fist — Keep first and second joints straight and gently bend third joint, as far as possible: gently straighten. 5-10 times as tolerated.
3. Fist — Bend all three joints gently, as much as possible: gently straighten. 5-10 times as tolerated.
4. Back — With hand flat on table, raise fingers toward ceiling; slowly return to table, 5–10 times as tolerated.

Example schedule:

Noon—Swelling management, exercises

3:00 p.m.—Scar massage, exercises

6:00 p.m.—Swelling management, exercises

9:00 p.m.—Scar massage, exercises

Appendix 1: Abbreviations

(A)	assisted, assistance
abd	abduction
ADL	activities of daily living
AFO	ankle-foot orthotics
AROM	active range of motion
ATNR	asymmetrical tonic neck reflex
(B)	both, bilateral
b.i.d.	twice a day
BKA	below knee amputee
c̄	with
c/o	complaints of
CHI	closed head injury
COTA	certified OT assistant
CT scan	computed tomography test
CVA	cerebrovascular accident
d/c	discharge
depend	dependent
DIP	distal interphalangeal
DJD	degenerative joint disease
DM	diabetes mellitus
doff	take off clothing
don	put on clothing
dx	diagnosis
ECG	electrocardiogram
EOM	edge-of-mat
ETOH	ethanol/alcohol
eval	evaluation, evaluate
ext	extension
F−	fair (40%)
F	fair (50%) or female (depending on text)
F+	fair (60%)
flex	flexion
fx	fracture

G–	good (70%)
G	good (80%)
G+	good (90%)
hemi	hemiplegia
hr	hour
hx	history
ICU	intensive care unit
IDDM	insulin-dependent diabetes mellitus
indep	independent
(L)	left
LE	lower extremity
LOS	length of stay
LTG	long-term goals
M	male
max	maximal
MI	myocardial infarction
min	minimal
MMT	manual muscle test
mod	moderate
MP	metacarpophalangeal joint
MS	multiple sclerosis
MVA	motor vehicle accident
MVPT	motor free visual perception test
N	normal
NG-tube	nasogastric tube
npo	nothing by mouth
nsg	nursing
od	once daily
OOB	out of bed
OT	occupational therapy
Ox or O_2	oxygen
P–	poor (10%)
P	poor (20%)
P+	poor (30%)

p.r.n. whenever necessary
para paraplegia
phys dys physical dysfunction
PIP proximal interphalangeal
PROM passive range of motion
pt patient
PT physical therapy
q.d. per day
(R) right
RA rheumatoid arthritis
rehab rehabilitation
s̄ without
s/p status post
SBA standby assistance
SP speech
STG short-term goals
STNR symmetrical tonic neck reflex
sup supination
T trace (5%)
THR total hip replacement
TR therapeutic recreation specialist
TTWB toe-touch weight bearing
tx treatment/treat or therapy
UE upper extremity
UTI urinary tract infection
w/c wheelchair
WBAT weight bearing as tolerated
WBQC wide-base quad cane
WFL within functional limits
wk week
y/o years old
y/n yes/no
yrs years

■ Appendix 2: Symbols

2°	secondary
→	to the right, or to or toward
←	to the left
↔	to the right and left, or to and from
✔	flexion
/	extension
#	pounds
↓	decreased or decrease
↑	increased or increase
x	times
x 1	times 1 (requires one person to assist)
x 2	times 2 (requires two people to assist)
0	zero (no contraction felt in the muscle)

C

Communication
- empathy, 20
- home program, 28–29
- listening skills, 19–20
- nonverbal, 19–20
- parameters, 19–20
- patient interview, 8
- treatment planning, 17–20

Community program, health care continuum, 25, 27–28

Cost of care, 7

D

Diagnosis, occupational therapy evaluation, 6, 7

Discharge process, 23–29
- health care continuum, 24–28

Documentation. See *Medical chart*

E

Empathy, 20

F

Facility type, occupational therapy evaluation, 6–7

H

Health care continuum, 24–28
- community program, 25, 27–28
- home health care, 25, 27
- hospital, 25, 26
- long-term care, 25, 26
- outpatient services, 25, 27
- progression patterns, 25
- reentry program, 25, 27
- rehabilitation, 25, 26–27

Home health care, health care continuum, 25, 27

Home program
- communication, 28–29
- components, 28
- development, 28–29
- purpose, 28
- types of information, 29

Hospital, health care continuum, 25, 26

I

Insurance reimbursement, medical chart, 2

L

Listening skills, communication, 19–20

Long-term care, health care continuum, 25, 26

Long-term goal, 4

M

Medical chart
- information relevance, 2–5
- information types, 3–4, 5
  - assessment, 4
  - objective, 3–4
  - plan, 4
  - subjective, 3
- insurance reimbursement, 2
- as legal document, 2–3
- occupational therapist review, 5
- student development, 2
- use by other professionals, 2
- usefulness, 2–3

Motivation, 17–18

N

Nurse, occupational therapy evaluation, 9–10

O

Occupational therapist, patient's emotions and, 18–19

Occupational therapy evaluation, 1–10
- case manager, 10
- diagnosis, 6
- facility type, 6
- factors, 5–7
- nurse, 10
- physical therapist, 9
- physician, 8–9
- recovery phase, 6
- registered dietitian, 9
- remuneration, 7
- social worker, 9
- speech–language pathologist, 9
- therapeutic recreation specialist, 9

Outpatient services, health care continuum, 25, 27

P

Patient interview, 8
  communication, 8
Physical therapist, occupational therapy evaluation, 8
Physician
  occupational therapy evaluation, 8
  as team leader, 8
Psychosocial aspects of health care, 18

R

Record keeping. See *Medical chart*
Recovery phase, occupational therapy evaluation, 6, 7
Reentry program, health care continuum, 25, 27
Referral, treatment planning, 13–14
Registered dietitian, occupational therapy evaluation, 9
Remuneration, 7

S

Short-term goal, 4
Social worker, occupational therapy evaluation, 9
Speech-language pathologist, occupational therapy
  evaluation, 9
Student development
  confusion phase, 12–13
  integration phase, 13
  medical chart, 2–3
  stagnation phase, 12
Symptom, patient interpretation of, 18–19

T

Therapeutic recreation specialist, occupational therapy
  evaluation, 9
Treatment goal
  functional area of focus, 15–16
  measurable end point, 15, 16–17
  purpose, 15
  treatment planning, 15–17
  use of verbs, 15
  writing effective, 15–17
Treatment planning, 11–20
  factors, 13–14
  patient's current situation, 14
  patient's current status, 14
  patient's goals, 14
  process, 14
  referral, 13–14
  student development, 12–13
  therapeutic methods, 14
  treatment goal, 15–17